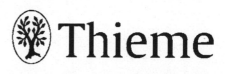

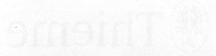

Robotic Gynecologic Surgery

Anupama Bahadur, DNB (Obstetrics and Gynecology), MNAMS
Professor
Department of Obstetrics and Gynecology
All India Institute of Medical Sciences
Rishikesh, Uttarakhand

Rajlaxmi Mundhra, MD, DNB (Obstetrics and Gynecology), MNAMS
Associate Professor
Department of Obstetrics and Gynaecology
All India Institute of Medical Sciences
Rishikesh, Uttarakhand

Padma Shri Prof. Ravi Kant, FAMS, FRCS (Edinburg), FRCS (England), FRCS (Glasgow), FRCS (Ireland), MS, DNB, FACS, FICS,
Dr. B. C. Roy (Eminent Medical Teacher)
Director and CEO
All India Institute of Medical Sciences
Rishikesh, Uttarakhand

Thieme
Delhi • Stuttgart • New York • Rio de Janeiro

Director—Medical Communications & Corporate Sales:
Dr Nitendra Sesodia
Director—Editorial Services: Rachna Sinha
Project Managers: Gaurav Prabhuzantye and
Shruti Kaushik
Vice President—Sales and Marketing: Arun Kumar Majji
Managing Director and CEO: Ajit Kohli

Thieme Medical and Scientific Publishers Private Limited
A 12, Second Floor, Sector 2, Noida 201 301,
Uttar Pradesh, India, +911204556600
Email: customerservice@thieme.in
www.thieme.in

Cover design: © Thieme
Cover image source: © Thieme

Page make-up by RECTO Graphics, India

Printed in India

5 4 3 2 1

ISBN 978-93-90553-87-7

Important note: Medicine is an ever-changing science undergoing continual development. Research and clinical experience are continually expanding our knowledge, in particular our knowledge of proper treatment and drug therapy. Insofar as this book mentions any dosage or application, readers may rest assured that the authors, editors, and publishers have made every effort to ensure that such references are in accordance with **the state of knowledge at the time of production of the book**.

Nevertheless, this does not involve, imply, or express any guarantee or responsibility on the part of the publishers in respect to any dosage instructions and forms of applications stated in the book. **Every user is requested to examine carefully** the manufacturers' leaflets accompanying each drug and to check, if necessary in consultation with a physician or specialist, whether the dosage schedules mentioned therein or the contraindications stated by the manufacturers differ from the statements made in the present book. Such examination is particularly important with drugs that are either rarely used or have been newly released in the market. Every dosage schedule or every form of application used is entirely at the user's own risk and responsibility. The authors and publishers request every user to report to the publishers any discrepancies or inaccuracies noticed. If errors in this work are found after publication, errata will be posted at www.thieme.com on the product description page.

Some of the product names, patents, and registered designs referred to in this book are in fact registered trademarks or proprietary names even though specific reference to this fact is not always made in the text. Therefore, the appearance of a name without designation as proprietary is not to be construed as a representation by the publisher that it is in the public domain.

This book, including all parts thereof, is legally protected by copyright. Any use, exploitation, or commercialization outside the narrow limits set by copyright legislation without the publisher's consent is illegal and liable to prosecution. This applies in particular to photostat reproduction, copying, mimeographing or duplication of any kind, translating, preparation of microfilms, and electronic data processing and storage.

Thieme addresses people of all gender identities equally. We encourage our authors to use gender-neutral or gender-equal expressions wherever the context allows.

Contents

Foreword

It is my privilege to write this foreword for this compendium edited by Anupama Bahadur, Rajlaxmi Mundhra, and Professor Ravi Kant. This title is timely as gynecological surgery has undergone a paradigm shift in the last few decades—from open access to laparoscopy, and now the robotic approach is gaining popularity and the indications for it is fast claiming the space once fully occupied by open surgery. The editors bring their combined experience and have done a commendable job by providing a unique insight into the evolution of robotic surgery in gynecology in a reader-friendly manner.

In the year 2010, when the Vattikuti Foundation launched its robotic surgery program in India, the surgical fraternity was skeptical about its value and sustenance in the Indian context. Capital cost of the equipment and the extraordinary laparoscopic skills of the Indian surgeons were the major hindrances in its initial take-off. It was considered an extravagant, worthless substitute to conventional laparoscopic surgery; but the same fraternity revised its opinion by transferring its surgical skills to robotic surgery. Following urology, gynecology is the fastest growing specialty, popularizing the use of robotics in benign as well as malignant conditions with excellent patient outcomes. This could only be achieved with the mentorship of Vattikuti international network of robotic surgeons who supported the foundation by traveling to India and putting their best in training the trainers. Now we have highly competent homegrown talent to disseminate robotic surgical skills and Anupama Bahadur is one example. I met her during a robotic surgery council meeting at Mussoorie while she was the lead team member to start a robotic surgery program at the All India Institute of Medical Sciences, Rishikesh, under the tutelage of the dynamic leadership of Professor Ravi Kant. Within a short span of time, with her endurance, she became an integral part of the Robotic Surgeons Council of India and has contributed significantly to the growth of robotic surgery in gynecology. Rajlaxmi worked relentlessly behind the scenes towards meeting this common goal.

Since the FDA approved da Vinci system for its gynecologic application, it had a phenomenal growth in the United States, growing at the rate of 30%. Besides its overall popularity in benign conditions, it proved its value in obese patients and in case of large uteri. Immediate patient outcomes in terms of decreased postoperative pain, greatly reduced need for postoperative pain killers, short hospital stay, reduced blood loss, and surgeon's preference are too significant to be ignored.

While the robotic surgery in general and gynecology in particular is on a growth spiral, this comprehensive, one-stop information source is very timely. It has handpicked subjects and the expertise of its long list of authors, and majority of the authors are the members of the founding team that developed robotic surgery in India. Besides the techniques to deal with different indications, this book includes possible complications of pelvic surgery such as ureteral injury, and gives surgical tips to avoid and effectively manage such injuries irrespective of the pathology the surgeon is dealing with.

This book is a compilation of all the relevant and updated information pertaining to robotic gynecologic surgery incorporating the in-depth knowledge and experience of established experts in robotic surgery. The target audience for this book includes gynecologists, urogynecologists, gynae-oncologists, and even patients who wish to understand the benefit of robotic-assisted surgery. The authors have presented in a concise manner the operative setup, instruments required, and surgical techniques with illustrated figures and photographs to supplement the text. The comprehensive videos that can be accessed through QR codes will help young surgeons learn from the experts and hone their surgical skills in robotics.

This book would be a necessary tool in the armamentarium of practicing gynecologists and trainees alike and for those who are desirous of keeping their surgical skills updated in an endeavor to give the best to their patients.

I thank the editors for their hard work and sincere attempt to push the boundaries of the specialty.

Mahendra Bhandari, MD, MBA
CEO Vattikuti Foundation;
Director Robotic Surgery Education and Research
Vattikuti Urology Institute
Henry Ford Hospital Detroit
Detroit, Michigan, USA

Preface

With the approval of da Vinci Robotic surgical system by FDA in 2005, its use in gynecological procedures has witnessed an exponential growth owing to both comfort of the surgeons and their ease of performing complex surgeries. Greater precision due to better visualization, shorter learning curve, ergonomic console designed to reduce fatigue, and camera control in the hands of the surgeon has expanded the horizon of gynecological surgeries for both benign and malignant cases—and for the patient, rapid postoperative recovery, shorter hospital stay, less blood loss, less pain, faster return to routine activities, and reduced morbidity.

Robotic surgery requires training of a surgeon for a unique set of surgical skills. The skill of the robotic surgeon mimics open surgery but with a computerized interface. With more hospitals being in the process of acquiring a robot, safe and standardized training of residents in this new technology is becoming important.

All the authors who have contributed are stalwarts in the field of robotics and have shared their rich clinical experience, surgical skills, and practical tips. The book aims to discuss the surgical aspects faced during robotic gynecological surgeries and is accompanied by videos which can be accessed through QR codes. The book addresses pertinent issues like cost-benefit analysis of robotic gynecological surgery, robotic versus laparoscopy for gynecological surgery, and even deals with complications of robotic gynecological surgery.

It is our endeavor to bring to you a book with relevant and up-to-date information in the field of robotic gynecology. We are hopeful that it will help budding gynecologists become skillful surgeons as robotic surgery is here to stay.

We express our sincere thanks to the team at Thieme, especially Dr Nitendra Sesodia and Ms Shruti Kaushik for grooming us through this remarkable journey of book publishing and discussing the minutest details during editing sessions which helped this book take its final form.

We dedicate this book to our parents, family, students, and patients who have kept their belief in us.

Anupama Bahadur, DNB (Obstetrics and Gynecology), MNAMS
Rajlaxmi Mundhra, MD, DNB (Obstetrics and Gynecology), MNAMS
Padma Shri Prof. Ravi Kant, FAMS, FRCS (Edinburg), FRCS (England),
FRCS (Glasgow), FRCS (Ireland), MS, DNB, FACS, FICS

Contributors

Amit Gupta, MS (General Surgery), FRCS (Edinburg), FRCS (Glasgow), MBA (Health Care Administration)
Professor
Department of Surgery
All India Institute of Medical Sciences
Rishikesh, Uttarakhand

Ankur Mittal, MS, MCh (Urology)
Associate Professor and Head
Department of Urology
All India Institute of Medical Sciences
Rishikesh, Uttarakhand

Anoosha K. Ravi, MS (Obstetrics and Gynecology), DNB
Senior Resident
Department of Obstetrics and Gynecology
All India Institute of Medical Sciences
Rishikesh, Uttarakhand

Anshumala Shukla Kulkarni, MD (Obstetrics and Gynecology), DGO, FCPS
Fellow in Minimally Invasive Surgery, Australia;
Consultant and Head
Minimal Access Gynecology;
Laparoscopic and Robotic Surgeon
Kokilaben Dhirubhai Ambani Hospital
Mumbai, Maharashtra

Anupama Bahadur, DNB (Obstetrics and Gynecology), MNAMS
Professor
Department of Obstetrics and Gynecology
All India Institute of Medical Sciences
Rishikesh, Uttarakhand

Anupama Rajanbabu, MD, MRCOG
Fellowship Gynecologic Oncology
Professor and Head
Department of Gynecologic Oncology
Amrita Institute of Medical Sciences
Kochi, Kerala

Bana Rupa, MD (Obstetrics and Gynecology)
Consultant Gynecology
Apollo Health City, Jubilee Hills
Hyderabad, Telangana

Bhavna Gupta, DA, DNB, MNAMS, FIPM, International fellow NIV (Spain), PDCR(Advanced)
Assistant Professor
Department of Anesthesiology
All India Institute of Medical Sciences
Rishikesh, Uttarakhand

Divya Mishra, MD (Obstetrics and Gynecology)
Fellow in Minimally Invasive Gynecology
Sunrise Hospital
Kochi, Kerala

Farhanul Huda, MS (General Surgery)
Additional Professor
Department of General Surgery
All India Institute of Medical Sciences
Rishikesh, Uttarakhand

Indira Sarin, DNB (Obstetrics and Gynecology)
Assistant Professor
Department of Obstetrics and Gynecology
NIMS Medical College
Jaipur, Rajasthan

Karthik Chandra Vallam, MCh (Surgical Oncology)
Consultant Surgical Oncologist and Robotic Surgeon
Apollo Cancer Hospital
Visakhapatnam, Andhra Pradesh

Madhavi Dokku, MS (Obstetrics and Gynecology), MCh (Gynecology)
Senior Resident
Department of Gynecology
Amrita Institute of Medical Sciences
Kochi, Kerala

Monica Gupta, MD (Obstetrics and Gynecology), DNB, MRCOG, DM (Reproductive Medicine)
Assistant Professor
Department of Obstetrics and Gynecology
All India Institute of Medical Sciences
New Delhi

Praveen Kumar, MS (General Surgery)
Assistant Professor
Department of Surgery
Himalayan Institute of Medical Sciences, Jolly Grant
Dehradun, Uttarakhand

Priya Kapoor, MS, DNB (Surgical Oncology)
Manipal Comprehensive Cancer Center
Manipal Hospital
Bengaluru, Karnataka

Rajkumar Kottayasamy Seenivasagam, MS, MCh, FRCS Ed, FACS
Associate Professor
Department of Surgical Oncology
All India Institute of Medical Sciences
Rishikesh, Uttarakhand

Rajlaxmi Mundhra, MD, DNB (Obstetrics and Gynecology), MNAMS
Associate Professor
Department of Obstetrics and Gynecology
All India Institute of Medical Sciences
Rishikesh, Uttarakhand

Reeta Mahey, MD (Obstetrics and Gynecology), DNB
Additional Professor
Department of Obstetrics and Gynecology
All India Institute of Medical Sciences
New Delhi

Rooma Sinha, MD (Obstetrics and Gynecology)
Honorary Professor Gynecology, Laparoscopic and Robotic Surgeon
Minimal Access and Robotic Surgery
Apollo Health City, Jubilee Hills
Hyderabad, Telangana

Shiv Charan Navriya, MS, MCh (Urology)
Assistant Professor
Department of Urology
All India Institute of Medical Sciences
Rishikesh, Uttarakhand

Shweta Shetye, DGO, DNB (Obstetrics and Gynecology)
Associate Consultant
Kokilaben Dhirubhai Ambani Hospital
Mumbai, Maharashtra

Somashekhar S.P., MS, MCh (Oncology), FRCS (Edinburg)
Chairman and Head of Department
Surgical Oncology MHEPL;
Consultant Surgical & Gynec. Onco & Robotic Surgeon, HIPEC Super Specialist
Manipal Comprehensive Cancer Center
Manipal Hospital
Bengaluru, Karnataka

Sunil Kumar, MS, MCh (Urology)
Assistant Professor
Department of Urology
All India Institute of Medical Sciences
Rishikesh, Uttarakhand

Utkarsh Kumar, MS (General Surgery)
Ex-Senior Resident
Department of Surgery
All India Institute of Medical Sciences
Rishikesh, Uttarakhand

1 da Vinci Robot: Machine and Instruments

Anupama Bahadur, Anoosha K. Ravi, and Rajlaxmi Mundhra

The future is already here! For almost two decades now, surgeons have been serviced by this ingenious machine called the da Vinci Robotic surgical system by Intuitive Surgical Systems Incorporation, Sunnyvale, CA. The surgical skill has been refined and promoted by this mechanical interface between the surgeon and the patient. All surgical fraternities, including gynecology, have embraced Robot-assisted laparoscopic surgeries. The first robot-assisted hysterectomy was done in 2001[1] at the University of Texas, which along with many other hysterectomies in the University of Michigan[2] provided the safety data and finally FDA approval in April 2005. Albeit few limitations, robot-assisted surgery is the inevitably preferred approach over conventional laparoscopy in minimally invasive surgery.

The Basis and Advancement

The history of robots dates back to the mechanical knight of Leonardo da Vinci from around the year 1495, which probably influenced the Intuitive Corporation to name this surgical system after him. "Robota" in Czech meaning "forced labor" aptly describes these machines which assist humans in mechanical work.

Two competitive systems shared the beginning years of robots in the surgical field; Zeus and da Vinci surgical systems. Zeus surgical system by Computer Motion promoted a voice-controlled endoscopic manipulator and attracted laparoscopic surgeons to improve precision. On the other hand, da Vinci surgical system was marketed toward open surgeons. The year 2003 was a landmark in robot-assisted surgery when Zeus and da Vinci's merger was announced, after which only da Vinci system prevailed.[3]

This surgical advancement has ever been evolving and what the future holds is nothing short of a miracle. The upcoming competitions like Senhance system, SPORT surgical system, Medrobotics, minirobots, and others hold a great promise in overcoming present limitations, with major attention on reducing the size of the machine, reducing the expenses, further improvising the flexibility of the instruments, improving dexterity, creating wireless modes, and providing haptic feedback.

da Vinci Surgical System

This surgical system has had six models: Standard, S, Si, Xi, X, and SP (chronologically).[4] Each has three subsystems, which are integrated:
1. Surgeon console.
2. Vision cart.
3. Patient side cart.

Surgeon Console

The surgeon console is away from the sterile field. It can be either single (**Fig. 1.1**) or dual (**Fig. 1.2**) like in Si system and beyond. The dual console is seated by the surgeon along with the co-surgeon or trainee.

Stereo Viewer

The surgeon views the surgical field as captured by the endoscope through a stereo viewer. The viewport supports the head and neck of the surgeon. Infrared sensors on both sides of the console sense the movement of the head and automatically deactivate the robotic arms when the head moves away from the view port, thus

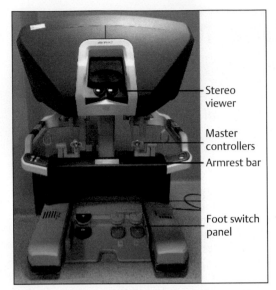

Fig. 1.1   Surgeon console.

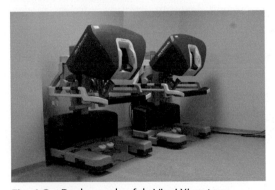

Fig. 1.2   Dual console of da Vinci Xi system.

avoiding any injuries. Much like the stereoscope, it has binocular vision. The image viewed is real-time, 3D, and of high resolution. The surgeon can also see system settings and alert messages on the screen.

It can have up to two additional images. TilePro function enables the surgeon to have a multi-input display which can be the 3D model of vascular anatomy or imaging of the affected area to help guide precise dissection and avoid complications.

Master Controllers

They are two in number, one for each hand. The thumb holds it, and the index/middle finger and the fingers are supported by Velcro straps. The endowrist instruments mimic the movements of the surgeon's hands on the master controller and apply those movements in the surgical field with a delay of not more than 150 ms.

The movements are intuitive, unlike the counterintuitive actions of conventional laparoscopy. The jaws of surgical instruments imitate the movements of fingers on master controller as seen in the stereo viewer. It is like the extension of surgeon's hand. The added benefit of tremor reduction improves the dexterity of the surgery in which the refinement can be up to 3:1.

Clutch feature: It is another safety mechanism to avoid unintended movement of the instruments. By pressing the gray button, the robotic arms are disengaged from that of the controllers to facilitate repositioning of the masters to a comfortable position. The feature is much like lifting the computer mouse.

Focus feature: The image on the stereo viewer is better focused by pressing and rotating the controller clockwise and anticlockwise like the way we do with camera head of the laparoscope.

Armrest Bar

This is the adjustable horizontal platform for the surgeon to rest his arms. It has two lateral pods and middle touchpad.

Floor Panel

There are three pedals on the left: One each for camera control, the primary clutch, and the control of arms swap. The pedals on the right are colored and used for applying electrosurgical energy.

The camera pedal, when pressed, engages the clutch for the instruments and switches the control to the camera arm. The movements of the controllers move the camera accordingly. This adjustment is similar to reading a newspaper held with both arms. Controllers move vertically above to see the caudal structure. Both controllers move to the right to know the structure on the left. Also, the controllers get nearer to the surgeon to advance the camera closer to the structure.

Toggle pedal: Among the four robotic arms, one is for the camera, and the other three are for instruments. It is not possible to control all three tools with two hands at the same time.

Hence, the toggle pedal helps to swap control between the fourth robotic instrument and the other as decided beforehand.

Clutch pedal: It functions similar to the clutch button on the controller—to disengage the instruments when there is a need to readjust the position of the master controller.

Vision Cart

It is a mobile tower hosting the touch screen monitor; an insufflator attached to CO_2 cylinder, an electrosurgical machine with an illuminator, an image and video recorder (**Fig. 1.3**).

Touch Screen Monitor

- It shows the real-time surgery as seen in the stereo viewer.
- It allows for telestration and hence communication with the patient side–assisting team and the surgeon on the console.
- It displays messages and alerts.
- It shows the number of uses of the particular instrument. Generally, the endowrist instruments should be replaced after 10 uses.[5]

Illuminator

Xenon light is provided by the illuminator which travels to the endoscope through the fiberoptic cable.

Patient Side Cart

This is a mobile tower with a robotic column and robotic arms (**Fig. 1.4**).

Mobilization and Placement

With earlier models such as Si system, the patient side cart needs to be repositioned depending on the change in the site of dissection. But with the novel gantry feature of the overhead boom in the Xi model, multiquadrant access is possible without moving the patient cart. The patient cart is transferred to the patient's side, left or right, with a motorized base. The steering handles with the throttles add to the ease of correct placement. Also, the laser light in the shape of "+" helps to centralize the overhead boom in pelvic surgeries (**Fig. 1.5**).

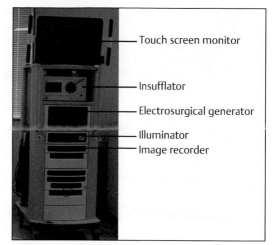

Fig. 1.3   Vision cart.

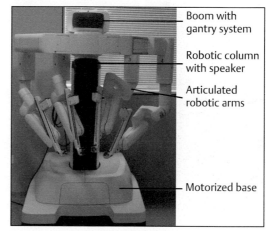

Fig. 1.4   Patient side cart.

Robotic Column

The robotic column is attached to four robotic arms. Each of them is numbered to enable selection for particular instruments. One of the robotic arms hosts the camera or the endoscope and it is called the camera arm. The other three robotic arms are for endowrist instruments. Positioning the robotic arms should be such that there is enough working space and no risk of collision.

Robotic Arms

Robotic arms have grooves and slots to house the instruments with complementary features, as

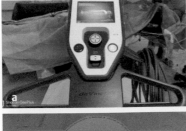

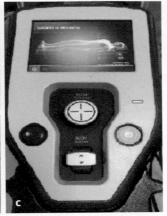

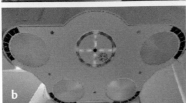

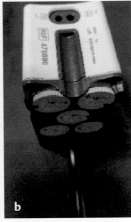

Fig. 1.5   **(a)** Steering handle with throttles. **(b)** Laser light on the boom to position the cart. **(c)** Control buttons to mobilize and position the patient side cart.

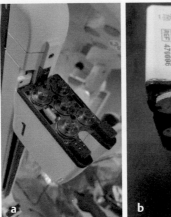

Fig. 1.6   **(a, b)** Fit between robotic arm and robotic instrument.

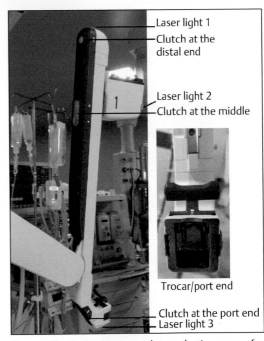

Laser light 1
Clutch at the distal end

Laser light 2
Clutch at the middle

Trocar/port end

Clutch at the port end
Laser light 3

Fig.   1.7   Features   on   the   robotic   arm   for mobilization and docking.

shown in **Fig. 1.6**. Some sounds suggest the right or wrong fit the assisting team should be familiar with. The clutches on the middle of the arm and at the port end helps in gross movement of the entire arm for easy connection to the robotic trocars (**Fig. 1.7**). The slot at the port end fits like a glove to the complementary knob on the robotic trocar. Laser lights on both ends indicate the function of the robotic arm.

Robotic arms move around a fixed pivot point. The trained assistant at the bedside helps insert, swap, or remove the robotic arms' robotic instruments. The button at the top of the robotic arm adjusts the trajectory of instruments into the cavity. It has a memory so that while reinserting, the instruments attain the same position as at the time of removal.

Targeting Feature

The laser targeting feature is present on the endoscope. After inserting into the peritoneal cavity, the endoscope points to an arbitrary middle point of the site of dissection. Upon pressing the targeting button for long, as shown in **Fig. 1.8**, the camera arm is fixed, and other arms automatically orient so that there is enough working space and no risk of collision.

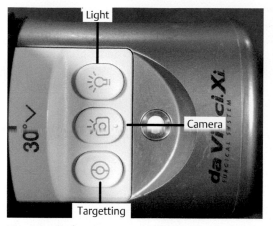

Fig. 1.8 Endoscope.

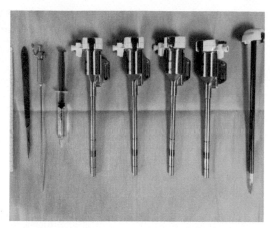

Fig. 1.9 Metal trocars, visiport, veress needle, marker, and ruler.

Robotic Trocars

These are 8-mm metal trocars inserted through the abdominal wall using either sharp or blunt obturators. The endoscope inserts through the visiport which has a transparent obturator tip (**Fig. 1.9**). These metal trocars can house 5- and 8-mm instruments. Robotic trocars should be placed at a minimum distance of 8 to 10 cm from one another to avoid collision of robotic arms. With the Xi model in pelvic surgeries, the trocars are placed in a straight line at or few inches above the umbilicus, depending on the size of the uterus or pelvic mass.

Robotic Instruments

Robotic instruments are endowrist instruments. They are so-called because of their articulated end, which is like that of the human wrist. It has seven degrees of motion which exceeds the range of the human wrist. The robotic instruments have long shafts, articulating wrist, and a movable tip (**Fig. 1.10**). Once mounted on the robotic arm, the system recognizes its function. They can be 5 or 8 mm in diameter. The robotic instruments with electrosurgical function have colored cables attached to the distal end: Green for monopolar and blue for bipolar.

Other instruments are staplers, vessel sealers, robotic irrigation, and suction cannula. The accessory or assistant port remains at least 5 cm away

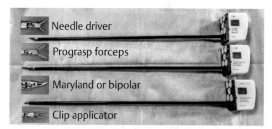

Needle driver

Prograsp forceps

Maryland or bipolar

Clip applicator

Fig. 1.10 Commonly used robotic instruments in gynecological surgeries.

from the robotic trocar. This port allows conventional laparoscopic instruments for retraction, clip application, suction, irrigation, and retrieval of specimens.

Firefly Technology

The knowledge of vascular and lymphatic anatomy is beneficial in oncology cases, requiring extensive dissection, including lymph node dissection. When injected into the blood vessel or the lymphatic vessel, Indocyanine green dye binds to the plasma proteins. It is capable of emitting an infrared signal when excited by laser light. This phenomenon is incorporated into the Si and Xi versions of the da Vinci surgical systems. The imaging equipment picks up the infrared signal and the precise vascular or lymphatic anatomy gets visible on the screen. This technology has been studied compared with conventional methods like methylene blue dye with the naked eye and Tc99 with gamma probe for sentinel lymph node dissection.

Single-Site Configuration

A five-lumen port can house an endoscope, two curved cannulae that cross at the level of the abdominal wall, an accessory port for 5- to 10-mm straight cannula, and an insufflation adaptor. The benefit is with the cosmesis as a single incision of 2 to 2.5 cm is sufficient. The Xi version can recognize this port, and the software reassigns the surgeon's hands with correct instruments.

Single Port or the SP System

Single-port system is the fourth-generation da Vinci surgical system. The technology holds a great potential with natural luminal surgeries like transoral and transanal. It has a single port of approximately 2.5 cm diameter. But unlike the single-site configuration, the cannulae are in parallel axes. The specialized articulated endoscope and instruments resemble snake-like movements, providing flexibility and the ability to easily manipulate spaces within confined spaces.

Evolution of da Vinci Surgical Systems and Their Key Features

da Vinci Standard System, 1999

- High-resolution 3D panoramic image.
- Four robotic arms.
- Endowrist instruments with seven degrees of freedom (DOF) and 90-degree articulation.
- Motion scaling and tremor reduction.
- High-resolution stereo viewer.
- It is no longer actively commercialized.

da Vinci S System, 2006

- 3D HD vision with 30% wider view and digital zoom feature to reduce instrument interference.

- 0- and 30-degree stereo endoscopes.
- Precise fingertip control with patented intuitive movements.
- Broad selection of 8 and 5 mm endowrist instruments.
- Faster docking with motorized patient cart, quick click cannula mounts.
- Single-use sterile adaptors with integrated drapes.
- Integrated touch screen monitor for team communication.
- TilePro multi-input display in the surgeon console screen.

da Vinci Si System, 2009

- Dual-console capability for training and collaboration.
- An updated user interface for streamlined setup.
- Extensibility for digital OR integration.

da Vinci Xi System, 2014

- Novel gantry system of the boom for multiquadrant access.
- Redesigned kinematics of patient cart for efficient deployment, roll-up, docking, and maximizing workspace.

da Vinci X, 2017

- Smaller and thinner arms.
- Laser guidance for a patient card for cart placement.
- Intuitive grab-and-move feature that simplifies docking.
- Affordable with the advanced technology of Xi system.

da Vinci SP

- Fourth-generation surgical system.
- A single 2.5-cm cannula with three fully wristed elbowed instruments.
- Fully wristed endoscope.
- The boom can rotate 360 degrees and also the instrument cluster can rotate over 360 degrees within the cannula and hence the accessibility to any site is immense.

Future

The robotic surgical systems and their progressing technologies have expanded the horizon of possibilities in the field of minimally invasive surgery. Everything imaginable and beyond imagination is becoming a reality with every passing day with this scientific boon. The possible areas of improvement in the present-day scenario are smaller instruments, lesser cost, smaller size, more dexterous, and faster rehabilitation time with lesser complications.

Haptic Feedback

A software update to the Xi version is in the development stage, overcoming the drawback of haptic feedback in the da Vinci surgical system. This advancement would allow surgeon to avoid arm collisions, improve the feel of structures, and reduce off-screen visceral injuries.

TransEnterix

TransEnterix by Senhance Surgical system has received FDA approval for gynecological surgeries. With new 3-mm instruments, this technology is evolving. The major advantage is that of cost containment. The system is characterized by an open console, polarized glasses for 3D display, eye tracking to move the camera, and haptic feedback similar to conventional laparoscopy.[6]

SPORT Surgical System

SPORT surgical system by Titan Medical is a versatile single incision system for single and multiquadrant surgeries. The system features multiarticulated instruments with single-use reusable tips. A single-arm mobile patient cart is easy to set up. The system is still under development and is not approved for use by FDA.[7]

Teleconsultation or Telesurgery

With the power of the Internet, it is possible to obtain teleconsultation or telesurgery as long as the relay delay is less than 150 ms. This advantage has found its usage in military surgery as well. The assistance can be cognitive and physical.

Minirobots

Minirobots are wireless devices that deploy within the abdominal cavity. With a camera and working arms, the device can reach the deepest of the cavities and perform precise surgery. This technology, which is in the making, will have a revolutionary effect on remote surgical care. Telesurgery with miniature robots is a field of active research.[8,9]

References

1. Diaz-Arrastia C, Jurnalov C, Gomez G, Townsend C Jr. Laparoscopic hysterectomy using a computer-enhanced surgical robot. Surg Endosc 2002;16(9):1271–1273
2. Reynolds RK, Advincula AP. Robot-assisted laparoscopic hysterectomy: technique and initial experience. Am J Surg 2006;191(4): 555–560
3. Lane T. A short history of robotic surgery. Ann R Coll Surg Engl 2018;100(6 suppl):5–7
4. So DM, Hanuschik M, Kreaden U. Chap. 7: The da Vinci surgical system. In: Rosen J, Hannaford B, Satava RM, eds. Surgical robotics: systems, applications, and visions. 1st ed. Springer; 2011
5. Bhandari A, Hemal A, Menon M. Instrumentation, sterilization, and preparation of robot. Indian J Urol 2005;21(2):83–85
6. Pappas T, Fernando A, Nathan M. Senhance surgical system: robotic-assisted digital laparoscopy for abdominal, pelvic, and thoracoscopic procedures. Handbook of robotic and image-guided surgery. 1st ed. Amsterdam, Netherlands: Elsevier; 2020:1–14
7. Titan Medical, Inc. Technology: http://titanmedicalinc.com/technology/ Accessed October 14, 2020
8. Rentschler ME, Platt SR, Berg K, Dumpert J, Oleynikov D, Farritor SM. Miniature in vivo robots for remote and harsh environments. IEEE Trans Inf Technol Biomed 2008;12(1): 66–75
9. Reichenbach M, Frederick T, Cubrich L, et al. Telesurgery with miniature robots to leverage surgical expertise in distributed expeditionary environments. Mil Med 2017;182(S1):316–321

2 Preoperative Preparation and Positioning for Robotic Gynecologic Surgery

Rooma Sinha and Bana Rupa

Introduction

Like any surgical procedure, patients must be appropriately prepared for robotic surgery before and during the operation. When compared to standard laparoscopic surgery, using the robotic platform requires modifications in the surgical preparation. An experienced surgical team ensures all essential steps in preparing a patient for surgery. The three crucial steps in achieving this are preoperative preparation of the patient, the operating room setup, and appropriate patient positioning.

Preoperative Preparation

Correct selection of patients regarding their indications and comorbidities should be considered before taking them for robotic surgery. One often tends to select patients with complex gynecologic problems for robotic surgery. Patients with comorbid medical conditions such as obesity and/or pulmonary, cerebral, vascular, cardiac, and ophthalmologic disorders (glaucoma) deserve particular attention. It is advisable that the respective specialist should appropriately evaluate these patients before undergoing robotic surgery. Like any surgical procedure, a detailed discussion and counseling about the advantages and disadvantages of robotic surgery should be done. Adequate information about the alternative forms of treatment should also be made available to patients before robotic surgery. Informed consent should be obtained. Appropriate preoperative blood investigations such as complete blood count, blood type, crossmatch, coagulation study, metabolic panel, chest X-ray, and electrocardiogram should be done.

Routine use of mechanical bowel preparation or nasogastric tube for better vision in surgery is not recommended.[1,2] However, we find the placement of nasogastric tube useful in large uteri where the primary port is being planned at Lee Huang's point close to the xiphisternum as this decompresses the stomach, reducing the risk of injury during port placement. Mechanical bowel preparation is only done in cases with advanced endometriosis where extensive adhesions to the bowel is expected. Intravenous cefazolin 1 g is our recommendation as prophylaxis for infection prevention, given 5 to 10 minutes before the induction of anesthesia. Deep vein thrombosis (DVT) prophylaxis should be considered in all patients undergoing robotic surgery. Although according to ACOG, individual and procedure-dependent risk factors should be taken into consideration for thromboprophylaxis, we recommend DVT prophylaxis in all patients undergoing robotic gynecologic surgery regardless of a patient's risk factor.[3] Intermittent pneumatic compression, as well as chemoprophylaxis with low-molecular-weight heparin, can be used.[4] Uterine manipulator is one of the most crucial part in preparation for any gynecologic surgery and is also true for robotic surgery. With its placement, the uterus can be moved inside the pelvis by the assistant, thus helping in dissection and coagulation, delineating the vaginal fornices, and reducing the risk of ureteral injuries. We use the RUMI Arch (Cooper Surgical) with the KOH colpotomizer during our robotic surgeries (**Fig. 2.1**). It offers a wide range of motion of the uterus; the KOH colpo-pneumooccluder minimizes air leak when the vaginal vault

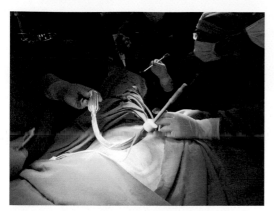

Fig. 2.1   Assembled RUMI arch.

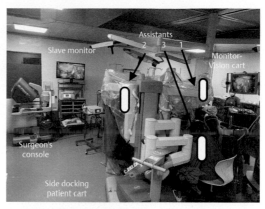

Fig. 2.2   Overview of the operation theatre.

is opened. Other uterine manipulators used are Clermont-Ferrand, which can move the uterus up to 140 angles in both anterior and posterior directions, and the Mangeshkar manipulator, which can shift the uterus in all directions with a wide range of motion.[5] However, one can use any manipulator that one is comfortable with.

Preparation of the Operating Room

Contrary to open or even laparoscopic surgery, robotic surgery is equipment-intensive. daVinci system has three components: A patient cart, vision tower, and surgeon's console. Care must be taken to provide ample space in the operating room to maneuver the equipment. We propose the room setup as shown in **Fig. 2.2**.

We usually position the patient cart on the right side of the patient. This is called "side docking," keeping the space between the legs free for uterine manipulation (**Fig. 2.3**). The vision cart is generally situated on the left side of the patient. The surgeon's console is located several feet from the operating table. The first assistant stands at the patient's left side, the second assistant at the patient's right side, and the third assistant between the stirrups. Each member of the team is assigned a role, and safe instrument exchange happens at the bedside with minimal assistance by the first assistant. Clear constant communication between the bedside assistants and the surgeon is essential for robotic surgery's safe progress.

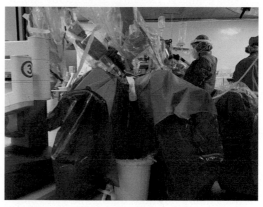

Fig. 2.3   Side docking of the patient cart on the right side of the patient. This ensures space between the legs for an assistant to manipulate the uterine manipulator.

Patient Positioning

Optimal patient positioning is essential for a successful robotic surgery procedure. It should provide adequate exposure of the pelvic structures as well as prevent any injury and complications in the patient. Robotic gynecologic procedures are focused on pelvis; hence, Trendelenburg position in the dorsal lithotomy position is essential. The Trendelenburg position itself can result in stretching or compression of nerves, leading to patients' nerve injury in the postoperative period.[6] Prolonged Trendelenburg position can increase risk of some unusual complications like corneal abrasion, cerebral edema, ischemic neuropathy, or laryngeal edema.[7] Lithotomy position does increase the risk of neuropathy in the lower limbs but abnormal positions of the arms can also result in the stretching of the brachial plexus. In fact, the brachial nerve injury complicates laparoscopic and robotic gynecologic surgery with an estimated incidence of 0.16%.[8] The nerves vulnerable to injury in the lower extremity during the lithotomy position are femoral, obturator, sciatic, lateral femoral cutaneous, and common peroneal nerves and can result in 0.03% motor deficits and 1.5% sensory deficits in the postoperative period.[6] The peroneal and saphenous nerves pass along the head of the fibula and medial tibial condyle, respectively. These should be protected by adequate padding to reduce injury. The surgical assistant should avoid leaning and applying their weight to prevent compression to nerves.

Modified lithotomy can be done with the help of adjustable leg support devices. The most common one used is Allen stirrups as they provide a good position for legs and protect legs and feet at pressure points (Allen Medical Systems, USA). These pneumatic stirrups are boot-shaped and can be attached to both sides of the operating room table (**Fig. 2.4**). One must ensure that both the stirrups are parallel to each other and at the same level.

It is recommended to put patients in extreme Trendelenburg positions during the gynecologic robotic surgery. This poses a problem of cephalad slipping of the patients. The rigid positioning of the robotic arms on the robotic trocars cannot accommodate this cephalad shift, resulting in a pull at the port site, potentially injuring the abdominal wall. A robotic side cart poses unique problems during patient positioning. The position of the patient should also allow unhindered movement of the robotic arms, allowing them full range of movements. The arms can hit against the legs of the patients. One must be vigilant to ensure that the arms do not mechanically injure the legs while the surgical procedure is in progress. An antiskid material is recommended to be used under the patient to prevent patient slipping. A modified dorsal lithotomy position is maintained at a minimal external hip rotation; hip flexion (thigh-trunk angle) is maintained between 100 and 170 degrees and never beyond 180 degrees. The knee flexion is usually maintained between 90 and 120 degrees with hip abduction less than 90 degrees (**Fig. 2.5**). The thighs should remain at or above the plane of the table and the level of the patient's knees should not be higher than that of abdomen to avoid collisions with the robotic arms. The main areas to pay attention is the posterior and lateral part of the legs to prevent nerve injury; this can be achieved predominantly by allowing the legs to rest on the heel by using the stirrups appropriately. The buttocks are positioned at 2 to 3 cm beyond the edge of the table for easy manipulation of uterine elevators.

We describe a technique for patient positioning in gynecologic surgery and do not use shoulder

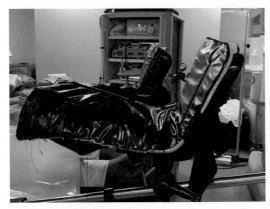

Fig. 2.4   Pneumatic stirrups.

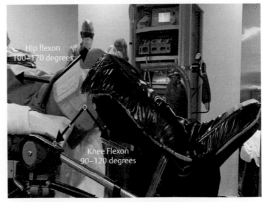

Fig. 2.5   Modified dorsal lithotomy with hips and knee flexion between 90 and 120 degrees. The abduction of thighs less than 90 degrees.

braces or straps. We use a draw sheet that is first placed horizontally on the table and then used to hold the patient by tucking the edges. The arms are tucked to the sides and not kept at an angle to the torso, which prevents brachial plexus injuries. Pads can be placed near elbows to reduce pressure on the ulnar nerve. The tucked patient's arm is kept in neutral position with the thumb pointing up and unclenched palms facing the thighs. Maintain the IV lines so that they are not obstructed while tucking the arms. When tucked on the sides, the collision between the robotic arms and the patient's arms can be prevented. Head should be stabilized in the midline position with the help of pads or foam. Use foam or cloth pad to protect the face from getting injured from the movements of the camera arm. Artificial tear drops are applied on the patient's eyes and the eyelids are closed with a simple tape to prevent undesired adverse effects such as corneal ulceration or injury (**Fig. 2.6**).

Prolonged Trendelenburg position can raise intraocular pressure and can lead to vision problems, ischemic optic neuropathy, and blindness.[9] It was generally considered that we need a steeper (>30 degrees) incline while performing robotic surgery when compared to traditional laparoscopy.[10,11] Such positions can increase risk of hemodynamic or ventilation difficulty, decrease in pulmonary compliance, and edema in the face, head, and neck. However with experience, we no longer use this extreme Trendelenburg position, enabling safe and feasible surgery without affecting the surgical exposure (**Fig. 2.7**). We use about 20- to 25-degree tilt for gynecologic robotic surgeries. Before the docking, we use the robotic telescope to visualize the whole abdomen and displace and tuck the small bowel and sigmoid colon from the operative field to the cephalic direction. The patient cart is then docked. Literature with smaller tilt have been reported, with a mean tilt angle of 28 degrees[12] and 16 degrees,[13] which completed gynecologic robotic procedures with adequate visualization in benign or malignancy pathology. When proper positioning is confirmed, the patient can be prepped and draped for the robotic surgical procedure.

Practical tips for positioning during robot-assisted benign gynecologic surgery:

- The arms should be tucked at the patient's sides, palm facing the thigh, and thumbs up.
- Position the head in the midline and cover with foam or cloth to prevent direct injury.
- Use an antislip mattress to prevent caudal slipping during Trendelenburg position.
- Modified lithotomy using pneumatic stirrups. Hip flexion (100–170 degrees) and knee flexion between 90 and 120 degrees, with hip abduction less than 90 degrees.
- Trendelenburg position tilt is between 20 and 30 degrees.

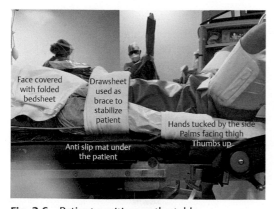

Fig. 2.6 Patient position on the table.

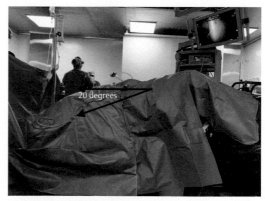

Fig. 2.7 Trendelenburg position; tilt 20 to 25 degrees.

References

1. Arnold A, Aitchison LP, Abbott J. Preoperative mechanical bowel preparation for abdominal, laparoscopic, and vaginal surgery: a systematic review. J Minim Invasive Gynecol 2015;22(5): 737–752

2. Kantartzis KL, Shepherd JP. The use of mechanical bowel preparation in laparoscopic gynecologic surgery: a decision analysis. Am J Obstet Gynecol 2015;213(5):721.e1–721.e5

3. Committee on Practice Bulletins–Gynecology, American College of Obstetricians and Gynecologists. ACOG Practice Bulletin No. 84: Prevention of deep vein thrombosis and pulmonary embolism. Obstet Gynecol 2007; 110(2 Pt 1):429–440

4. Feng JP, Xiong YT, Fan ZQ, Yan LJ, Wang JY, Gu ZJ. Efficacy of intermittent pneumatic compression for venous thromboembolism prophylaxis in patients undergoing gynecologic surgery: a systematic review and meta-analysis. Oncotarget 2017;8(12):20371–20379

5. Mettler L, Nikam YA. A comparative survey of various uterine manipulators used in operative laparoscopy. Gynecol Surg 2006;3(4):239–243

6. Warner MA, Warner DO, Harper CM, Schroeder DR, Maxson PM. Lower extremity neuropathies associated with lithotomy positions. Anesthesiology 2000;93(4):938–942

7. Gainsburg DM. Anesthetic concerns for robotic-assisted laparoscopic radical prostatectomy. Minerva Anesthesiol 2012;78(5):596–604

8. Shveiky D, Aseff JN, Iglesia CB. Brachial plexus injury after laparoscopic and robotic surgery. J Minim Invasive Gynecol 2010;17(4):414–420

9. Molloy BL. Implications for postoperative visual loss: steep Trendelenburg position and effects on intraocular pressure. AANA J 2011; 79(2):115–121

10. Boggess JF, Gehrig PA, Cantrell L, et al. Perioperative outcomes of robotically assisted hysterectomy for benign cases with complex pathology. Obstet Gynecol 2009;114(3): 585–593

11. Geppert B, Lönnerfors C, Persson J. Robot-assisted laparoscopic hysterectomy in obese and morbidly obese women: surgical technique and comparison with open surgery. Acta Obstet Gynecol Scand 2011;90(11):1210–1217

12. Gould C, Cull T, Wu YX, Osmundsen B. Blinded measure of Trendelenburg angle in pelvic robotic surgery. J Minim Invasive Gynecol 2012;19(4):465–468

13. Ghomi A, Kramer C, Askari R, Chavan NR, Einarsson JI. Trendelenburg position in gynecologic robotic-assisted surgery. J Minim Invasive Gynecol 2012;19(4):485–489

3 Anesthetic Considerations in Robotic Gynecologic Surgeries

Bhavna Gupta

Abstract

Capek and his colleagues introduced the word "Robot" in Rossum's *Universal Robots*, unveiled in the year 1921.[1] A robot is a *"computer-controlled manipulator with an automated sensor that can be remotely controlled to shift and position tools to perform a wide variety of tasks."* The surgical robot is a computer-assisted, preprogrammed, system regulated by a surgeon. Dr. James, Geof Auchinleck, and Dr. Brain Day used the first surgical robot in Vancouver in 1983.[2] Initial procedures were done on dogs and later in human patients. da Vinci system was the first robotic system approved by the Food and Drug Approval (FDA) for intra-abdominal surgeries in the United States. Robotic gynecologic surgery received FDA approval in 2005.[2] The concept behind automation systems is that the system translocates the surgeon to the operation site and allows ergonomic three-dimensional perception of the console. Robots are commonly used in almost all surgical fields, including vascular, thoracic, gynecologic, urologic, orthopaedic, general, and pediatric surgery. Robotic surgery is popular owing to decreased blood loss, reduced postoperative pain, shorter hospital stays, and improved visualization of delicate structures. This chapter focuses on clinical issues for anesthesiologists in the management of patients undergoing gynecologic robotic surgery.

Literature Review

A comprehensive search of multiple databases including PubMed, Cochrane Databases of Systematic Reviews, Scopus, EMBASE, Google, and Google Scholar was conducted for studies between 1990 and 2020, using the following words as the primary keys, either single or in different combinations: "anesthesia," "robotic surgery," "gynecologic," perioperative "management," "complications". References to the relevant papers were cross-checked, and the search queries were then analyzed by title and abstract for importance, with a priority for more relevant documents.

Introduction

Robotic-assisted laparoscopic surgery is a technologically advanced technique in gynecologic surgery. Robotic-assisted laparoscopic surgery was designed to overcome the problems faced by conventional laparoscopic techniques. One of the first gynecologic surgeries conducted with da Vinci system was the reanastomosis of tubes. Gynecologic procedures are conducted in a small area, (i.e., pelvis, and traditional laparoscopic techniques limit the degree of freedom of movement); thus, robotic procedures lead to ease in the performance of complex tasks. Various robotic gynecologic procedures include lymph node dissection, tubal reanastomosis, myomectomy, hysterectomy, sacral colpopexy, retroperitoneal ectopic pregnancy, and ovarian cystectomy.[1-3] An anesthesiologist's various concerns while conducting a robotic gynecologic procedure include a steep head low position, difficult access to the patient after docking, impact of pneumoperitoneum, and surgical duration.[4-7] Critical aspects of successful general anesthesia include: Evaluating the patient's comorbidities, understanding the risk associated with robotic equipment, and placing the patient with caution.

The significant benefits of laparoscopic robotic surgery are multifactorial, with shortened recovery time being the significant desirable benefit. The laparoscopic approach reduces the manipulation of bowel and peritoneum, resulting in a significantly reduced incidence of paralytic ileus in the postoperative period. Enteral nutrition is resumed rapidly as compared to open procedures, limiting the requirement of intravenous fluids, which indirectly is associated with poor wound repair, tissue wall edema, and prolonged postoperative recovery. Small incisions are made in the abdomen instead of large incisions, as seen in open procedures, thereby reducing postoperative pain, less opioid requirement, early recovery from surgery and anesthesia, and rapid wound healing. These benefits are particularly significant in obese patients, as open procedures are technically more challenging, associated with an increased incidence of bleeding, postoperative pain, and delayed recovery. The various advantages and disadvantages are summarized in **Fig. 3.1**.

Laparoscopic surgical procedures are traditionally contraindicated in severe ischemic heart disease, significant renal dysfunction, end-stage respiratory disease, etc. However, the risk to the particular patient for a specific laparoscopic procedure must be balanced between the risk of complications due to the proximity, time, magnitude of CO_2 absorption (CO_2), and physiological effects of pneumoperitoneum and the reduced postoperative recovery period that may outweigh the increased intraoperative risk. Universally acknowledged contraindications include preexisting elevated intracranial pressure, significant uncorrected hypovolemia, and those with existing right-to-left cardiac shunts or patent foramen ovale. The benefits of robotic surgical procedures should be weighed against risk on an individualistic basis.

Preoperative Assessment

A standard preanesthetic evaluation is essential to recognize any comorbidities, obesity, and elderly age. It is necessary to enquire specifically about pulmonary or cardiac risk factors. The surgical procedure includes a steep positioning of Trendelenburg, along with pneumoperitoneum, which can lead to considerable physiological fluctuations, as discussed in **Table 3.1** and **Fig. 3.2**. Any patient with significant respiratory or cardiovascular disease should be considered for the standard open surgical procedure or offered alternative nonsurgical modality.[2,4,5,8]

Advantages	Disadvantages
3-dimensional movement	Increased time required for docking and undocking of the Robot
Easier access to inaccessible surgical areas	Absence of tactile feedback
Faster recovery	The staff needs to be trained to rapidly de-dock, in case of an emergency.
A shorter length of stay	Rapid access to the patient is difficult
Better field of vision	Increased cost of surgery
Reduced pain	Bulkiness of robotic system
Especially useful for obese	
Ability to perform finer and tremor-free dissection	

Fig. 3.1   Advantages and disadvantages of robotic surgery over general surgery.

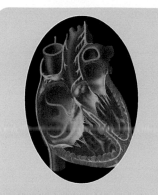
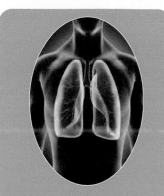
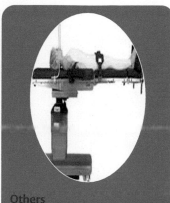

Cardiovascular
- Hypotension
- Hypertension
- Arrhythmia
- Increase in central venous pressure (CVP)
- Bradycardia
- Decrease in cardiac index (CI)
- Increase in systemic vascular resistance (SVR)

Respiratory
- Decrease in lung compliance
- Pneumothorax
- Subcutaneous emphysema
- Capnothorax
- Decrease in functional residual capacity (FRC)
- Hypercarbia
- Hypoxia

Others
- Peripheral nerve injury
- Plexus injury
- Airway, facial and brain edema
- Vascular, bowel and bladder injury
- Compartment syndrome
- Catecholamine secretion
- Increase in RAS activation

Fig. 3.2   Effects on various organ systems.

Table 3.1   Effects of surgery, positioning, and various organ effects

Surgical risks	• There is often a risk for damage to the solid viscera, blood vessels, intestines, or bladder due to the insertion of trocars in the abdominal cavity. • Venous gas embolism (VGE) may be caused by secondary trocar insertion in a blood vessel or by inadvertent inflation of a strong organ and may result in a catastrophic circulatory failure.
Positioning[8–11]	• Robotic gynecological procedures are carried in steep Trendelenburg position to visualize lower abdomen and pelvis. • There is always a risk of movement on the table; therefore, meticulous attention should be paid to ensure that vulnerable pressure points and eyes are covered to avoid injury.
Steep head low	• Prolonged steep Trendelenburg location is often correlated with the possibility of cerebral edema, facial edema, and upper airway edema. • There is a cephalic movement of the lung due to diaphragm displacement; thus, functional residual capacity and ventilation and perfusion mismatch are worsened; this is imperative in patients with impaired respiration or morbidly obese.

(Continued)

Table 3.1   *(Continued)* **Effects of surgery, positioning, and various organ effects**

Pneumoperitoneum[8–11]	• Pneumo means air, the presence of air in the peritoneal cavity is pneumoperitoneum for the visualization of organs. • While carbon dioxide (CO_2) is the agent of choice, other gases, including helium, argon, nitrous oxide, and oxygen, are often used to provide pneumoperitoneum, and have also associated problems such as combustion, intravascular insufflation, embolism, etc.
Cardiovascular effects[8–11]	• There is *a decrease in cardiac output and increased left ventricular filling pressure* secondary to a steep head low position. • *Systemic vascular resistance (SVR) increases* as intra-abdominal pressure is increased, secondary to aorta's mechanical compression and activation of renin-angiotensin axis. • *Mean arterial pressure also increases*, whereas renal, splanchnic, and portal flows decrease. • Compression of the inferior vena cava reduces preload and may lead to a *decrease in cardiac output* and subsequent reduction of arterial pressure, mainly if the patient is hypovolemic, which can be exacerbated secondary to cephalad displacement of the diaphragm. • Rise in intrathoracic pressure can also reduce blood flow through inferior vena cava.
Respiratory effects[11]	• Steep head low position also causes changes in respiration. • Diaphragmatic excursion is limited secondary to pneumoperitoneum, resulting in a rise in intrathoracic pressure, which leads to reduced *functional residual capacity and pulmonary compliance*. • All these lead to *pulmonary atelectasis, mismatch in ventilation and perfusion (V/Q) and hypoxemia*. • Absorbed CO_2 itself can cause *hypercarbia* during surgery.
Splanchnic effects	• A decrease in splanchnic and intestinal blood flow by up to 40% and a decrease in glomerular filtration rate (GFR) by 25% is analogous to an increase in intra-abdominal pressure. • It is related to a decline in cardiac performance, activation of compressive effects and neurohumoral factors, and the RAS pathway.
Neurological effects	• There *is an increase in intracerebral pressure* secondary to rise in intra-abdominal pressure secondary to raised intrathoracic pressure which cause limitation in cerebral venous drainage. • Though cerebral perfusion pressure (CPP) is well maintained by increase in MAP, but the rise in intracranial pressure can lead to *cerebral edema*. • There may be *temporary neurological dysfunction* that patients often experience on emergence, particularly those requiring extended periods of steep head low position.
Hypothermia[9–11]	• *Secondary to long surgery, exposure, cold intravenous fluids, respiratory gases, and CO_2 insufflation*
Restricted access	• Restricted access to the patient after the *massive Robot* is docked and draped, and even in a crisis, the process may be tasking even for defibrillation to heart.
Communication	• The Robot's efficient use to assist in surgery depends on the excellent coordination with all the theater team members.

The patient's height and weight should be carefully considered, as body mass index (BMI) more than 30 may be associated with difficult intubation, delayed gastric emptying, difficult vascular access, associated comorbidities, such as diabetes and hypertension History of obstructive sleep apnea should also be sought in case the patient is morbidly obese. Cardiovascular risk is assessed by a patient's symptoms, clinical examination, medications, and exercise tolerance. Current American Heart Association/American College of Cardiology (AHA/ACC) guidelines should be followed to determine whether the patient needs to be optimized before surgery. Patients with cardiac stents should be examined by a cardiologist before robotic gynecologic surgery, since the risk of surgical bleeding with anticoagulation medication needs to be balanced against the risk of stent thrombosis.

Patients with pulmonary disease should be screened for a history of smoke exposure (e.g., *Chula*) in addition to assessment of pulmonary dysfunction symptoms. Patients with asthma and chronic obstructive pulmonary disease should continue taking their inhalers and medications as prescribed by a pulmonologist. Similarly, renal insufficiency will likely be exacerbated by robotic surgery due to mechanical obstruction, patient positioning, and fluid restrictions, and therefore care must be taken to optimize renal function preoperatively.

At a minimum, preoperative studies for robotic gynecologic surgery should include an electrocardiogram, chest radiograph, blood counts, coagulation status, renal function, and electrolytes. The patient's blood should be typed and screened for particular antigens. Fasting blood glucose is required before surgery for diabetics. Prophylactic reflux medications in the form of nonparticulate antacids, antibiotics within 60 minutes of surgical incision and deep vein thrombosis prophylaxis with subcutaneous heparin, and sequential compression devices should be considered.

Perioperative Management

American Society of Anesthesiologists Monitoring

The impact of pneumoperitoneum and steep head low positioning on the respiratory system can be monitored using pulse oximetry and carbon dioxide end-tidal monitoring. Modern anesthesia workstation shows the information on peak airway pressures, plateau pressures, delivered tidal volumes, and complex flow-volume loops. Normocarbia should be preserved in order to preserve cerebrovascular homeostasis. Invasive arterial monitoring may be needed in patients with cardiovascular comorbidity. Esophageal Doppler Monitor (Lithium Dilution Cardiac Output Monitor) can provide more accurate preload assessment. Hemodynamic instability is better handled by optimizing preloading with fluid and judicious usage of vasoactive drugs. The routine and advanced American Society of Anesthesiologists (ASA) standard of monitoring are summarized in **Table 3.2**.

All robotic gynecologic procedures are nearly performed under general anesthesia with endotracheal intubation and neuromuscular blockade. Once the procedure starts, there is limited access to the patient. Therefore, all standard monitors are meticulously placed and secured. It is imperative to ascertain the functional intravenous line with additional tubings. These should all be checked and obtained before moving and positioning the patient. Endotracheal tube positioning must be tested frequently, as there is the possibility of endobronchial intubation and airway obstruction subsequent to tube migration resulting from diaphragm movement and pneumoperitoneum insufflation. There is limited access to the patient once the Robot is docked; thus, accidental patient movement during surgery can cause significant injury due to relatively immobile robotic arms accessing the patient.

Consequently, neuromuscular blockade should be optimal to maintain patient immobility during the procedure. In emergent situations such as cardiac arrest or a lost airway, the Robot will have to be moved to allow intervention and resuscitation access. Creating an emergency plan for moving the Robot should be discussed and agreed upon before every anesthetic induction. The various anesthetic considerations are summarized in **Table 3.3**.

General Anesthesia

General anesthesia (GA) is induced by intravenous route with opioids, usually fentanyl (2 µg/kg) and either propofol or thiopentone or etomidate or ketamine induction agent.

Table 3.2   Routine intra operative standard monitoring include

- Electrocardiograph (ECG)
- Non invasive blood pressure (NIBP)
- End tidal carbon dioxide (EtCO$_2$)
- Peripheral saturation (SpO$_2$)
- Additional monitors: Temperature, neuromuscular monitoring, urine output, bis-spectral index, invasive blood pressure monitoring, esophageal Doppler and cardiac output monitoring

Table 3.3   Anesthesia considerations in robotic assisted gynaecological surgery

Issues	Description	Anesthesia implications
Patient positioning	Steep Trendelenburg 25 to 45 degrees head down	• Compromised-hemodynamic • Compromised oxygenation • Restricted access to airway • Nerve injury
Pneumoperitoneum	CO$_2$ insufflation of peritoneum or thorax often for prolonged period	• Increased peak pressure • Increased plateau airway pressure • Decreased lung compliance and vital capacity • Atelectasis • Risk of pulmonary embolism • Hypotension
Hypothermia	Secondary to exposure, prolonged duration of surgery, fluids, surface area	• Infection • Bleeding • Cardiac events • Changes in drug metabolism • Patient discomfort • Increased length of stay
Restricted access	Because of bulky robotic instruments	• Emergency crisis situation may develop

The maintenance anesthesia is provided with oxygen-air/nitrous oxide and isoflurane or sevoflurane as inhalational agent. Desflurane is preferred in obese subsets, because of its rapid recovery. Neuromuscular blockade can either be achieved with vecuronium, rocuronium, or atracurium. An oxford pillow or head ring and a difficult intubation trolley should be available during induction. Anesthesia workstation, suction apparatus, and all airway equipment required for intubation are checked beforehand. Intubation is carried out in slight head-up position, and endotracheal tube position is checked by auscultation before handing over to surgeons (**Fig. 3.3**).

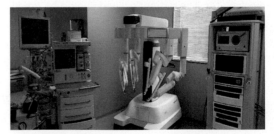

Fig. 3.3 A real picture of our Robotic Operation theater at level 6, AIIMS, Rishikesh, depicting Anesthesia Workstation and da Vinci Robot Surgical System. Photo provided courtesy of Dr. Kantha Manasa, Junior Resident in Department of Anaesthesiology.

Airway

The positioning of a cuffed endotracheal tube with optimum relaxation and positive pressure ventilation is standard practice. Endotracheal intubation protects against gastric aspiration and enables optimum regulation of CO_2 during surgery. The use of supraglottic airways, such as laryngeal mask airways, is associated with an increased risk of aspiration; thus, the use of supraglottic airways is controversial, particularly when there is a risk of longer duration of surgery.[4]

Ventilation

Steep positioning, cephalic movement of the diaphragm, and pneumoperitoneum may be associated with inadequate ventilation during laparoscopic robotic surgery. Conventional methods for delivering constant preset tidal volume and respiratory rate are associated with increased risk of barotrauma, especially in obese patients. As a result, pressure-controlled ventilation mode with titrated positive end-expiratory pressure (PEEP) offering higher instantaneous flow peaks minimizes peak pressures and enhances alveolar recruitment. Oxygenation is the preferred mode of ventilation.[5]

Analgesia

Since it is a minimally invasive surgery, pain is often short yet intense in up to 75% subsets, and requires opioids in the perioperative period. Regional techniques are increasingly being employed in robotic gynecologic surgery to spare opioids. Wound infiltration is also a helpful modality and reduces postoperative pain. Dexamethasone is also used as an analgesic agent and given just after induction.[6]

Fluid Management

Fluid management is balanced against a risk to minimize laryngeal and conjunctival edema. Most intravenous fluids should be administered within the last 30 minutes after Trendelenburg steep position has been changed. Loss of blood is negligible, and blood transfusion is rarely needed.

Emergence from Anesthesia

Neuromuscular block needs to be reversed with reversal agents including neostigmine and glycopyrrolate, after the patient starts taking their own spontaneous efforts. The trachea should not be extubated in case of suspected laryngeal edema, and larynx examination before extubation may be warranted. Some concern has also been raised for cerebral edema secondary to steep head low position for prolonged duration of time; therefore, it is imperative to check whether the patient is well awake and responding to commands appropriately at the time of extubation.

Considerations in Postoperative Area

The postoperative period is generally uneventful. All patients should receive additional oxygen during recovery to offset the effect of pneumoperitoneum on pulmonary function. The complications are negligible; the most common is ileus subsequent to pelvic hematoma and anastomosis leakage. Complications identified after robotic surgery can range from corneal abrasions, neuropathy, abdominal discomfort, bowel injury, and paralytic ileus. Blood transfusion is not usually needed. It is essential to prescribe multimodal analgesic agents, including acetaminophen and nonsteroidal anti-inflammatory drugs (if no contraindications exist). Few patients need pain-relief opioids. Before leaving the hospital, surgical drains must be removed and the patient must be mobile, afebrile, comfortable with oral pain killers, and must have passed urine, flatus, and/or feces.

Conclusion

Robotic surgery is a commonplace in gynecology and both anesthesiologist and gynecologist need to be well versed with the physiology, specialty's concerns, patient's comorbidities, their optimization, and risk and benefits on an individual basis; in doing so, patient outcome and satisfaction will continue to increase. Collaboration and coordination among surgeons, nurses, and anesthesiologists are essential in reducing risks and providing better surgical conditions and clinical outcomes.

References

1. Bush SH, Apte SM. Robotic-assisted surgery in gynecological oncology. Cancer Contr 2015; 22(3):307–313
2. Pilka R. Robotic surgery in gynecology. Rozhl Chir 2017;96(2):54–62
3. Park JY, Nam JH. Role of robotic surgery in cervical malignancy. Best Pract Res Clin Obstet Gynaecol 2017;45:60–73
4. Badawy M, Béïque F, Al-Halal H, et al. Anesthesia considerations for robotic surgery in gynecologic oncology. J Robot Surg 2011; 5(4):235–239
5. Gupta K, Mehta Y, Sarin Jolly A, Khanna S. Anaesthesia for robotic gynaecological surgery. Anaesth Intensive Care 2012;40(4):614–621
6. Kaye AD, Vadivelu N, Ahuja N, Mitra S, Silasi D, Urman RD. Anesthetic considerations in robotic-assisted gynecologic surgery. Ochsner J 2013;13(4):517–524
7. Mishra P, Gupta B, Nath A. Anesthetic considerations and goals in robotic pediatric surgery: a narrative review. J Anesth 2020;34(2):286–293
8. Chen K, Wang L, Wang Q, et al. Effects of pneumoperitoneum and steep Trendelenburg position on cerebral hemodynamics during robotic-assisted laparoscopic radical prostatectomy: a randomized controlled study. Medicine (Baltimore) 2019;98(21):e15794
9. Mishra P, Gupta B. Delayed reversal—hypothermia despite caution in a case of pediatric robotic pyeloplasty. J Neonatol Clin Pediatr. 2020;7:52
10. Berger JS, Alshaeri T, Lukula D, Dangerfield P. Anesthetic considerations for robot-assisted gynecologic and urology surgery. J Anesth Clin Res 2013;4:345
11. Sadashivaiah J, Ahmed D, Gul N. Anaesthetic management of robotic-assisted gynaecology surgery in the morbidly obese: a case series of 46 patients in a UK university teaching hospital. Indian J Anaesth 2018;62(6):443–448

4 Robotic Simple Hysterectomy

Rajlaxmi Mundhra and Anupama Bahadur

Abstract

This chapter discusses the indications and steps of robotic simple hysterectomy. Despite having a dearth of evidence regarding the benefits of robotic surgery compared to conventional laparoscopy for benign gynecologic pathologies, this mode of surgery has seen exponential growth in its indications in recent years.

Background

Hysterectomy is one of the most commonly performed gynecological procedures. The mode of surgery can be vaginal, laparotomy, laparoscopic, or robotic. The American Congress of Obstetricians and Gynaecologists (ACOG) considers vaginal route to be the most preferred method for patients undergoing benign hysterectomy and laparoscopic route may be considered when vaginal approach is not feasible.[1] Each surgical route has its complication rate and postoperative recovery time. Benefits of minimally invasive compared to open route have been seen in several studies. A recent Cochrane Database Systematic Review (2015) compared the four different surgical approaches of benign hysterectomy (abdominal, vaginal, laparoscopic, and robotic) in terms of effectiveness and safety.[2] The authors concluded that the vaginal route is superior to both the laparoscopic and abdominal routes in terms of faster return to normal activities. There was no difference in terms of primary outcome between laparoscopic and robotic hysterectomy.

In recent years, the robotic approach has seen exponential growth in various clinical specialties, including gynecology. Though current evidence suggests no major difference between robotic and laparoscopic hysterectomy, robotic surgery is a step ahead, having certain advantages and disadvantages as compared to conventional laparoscopy.

Benefits of Robotic Approach

- Robotic surgery gives a stable and fixed view of the surgical field as the camera control is directly under the control of the robotic surgeon compared to conventional laparoscopy. There is a constant change in visualizing the surgical field depending on patients' breathing and assistants' hand-eye coordination.[3]
- In robotic surgery, the instruments move in the same direction as the operating surgeon whereas in conventional laparoscopy, the movements are counterintuitive.
- Endowrist technology makes complex surgeries to be performed with the same ease as in open surgeries. These instruments have seven degrees of freedom and a motion similar to that of a human hand.
- Robotic surgery has a faster learning curve.
- Suturing is less tiring in the robotic approach. In conventional laparoscopy, long instruments enter the abdomen through a fixed point, thereby increasing the tendency to cause tremors and early fatigue among operating surgeons.

Disadvantages of Robotic Surgery

- The major disadvantage is the cost of surgery which remains the most prohibitive factor in its uptake.[4]
- A robotic surgeon too needs assistance in terms of change or cleaning of instruments during surgery.
- There is no tactile sensation of tissues for a robotic surgeon, leading to less secured surgical knots and increased tissue damage.[5]

Indications of Hysterectomy

Diaz-Arrastia et al performed the first robotic hysterectomy in 2002.[6] Robotic hysterectomy now finds its way in a broad spectrum of benign pathologies like leiomyoma, abnormal uterine bleeding, adnexal masses, and various other causes. Its use is increasing in staging of endometrial cancer. Data regarding its use in ovarian malignancies is limited and further randomized controlled trials and systematic reviews need to be undertaken to determine its oncological safety.

Technique

Port Placement and Docking

The patient should be in a dorsal lithotomy position with arms securely tucked at her sides.

Padded shoulder blades must be put. The patient should be in Trendelenburg position and incidences of corneal abrasion, corneal edema, and posterior ischemic optic neuropathy have been reported with prolonged positioning.[7] The latest robot model, da Vinci Xi, has four 8-mm identical arms, facilitating the exchange of cameras and instruments as and when required.

The port markings should be more or less in a straight or slightly curvilinear fashion (**Fig. 4.1**). The endoscope port is the first port and should be approximately 20 cm above pubic symphysis or 8 to 10 cm above the uterine fundus. There should be an 8 cm gap between each port marking. A gap of at least 2 cm should be there between any port and bony prominence. Through left-side port, bipolar forceps is introduced and a monopolar scissor is put through right-side port. Additional assistant ports are placed depending on the need for surgery.

Once port marking is completed, docking needs to be done. Side docking ensures better vaginal access for uterine manipulation and easy specimen retrieval.

Operating Steps

- Inspection of the entire abdominal cavity is the first step.
- The uterus remains elevated through the manipulator.
- The round ligament is clamped, cauterized, and cut (**Fig. 4.2**). The anterior leaf of broad ligament is incised to open the uterovesical fold of peritoneal reflection.

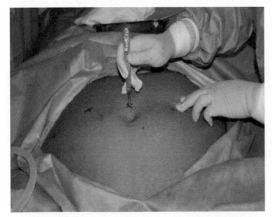

Fig. 4.1   Port markings.

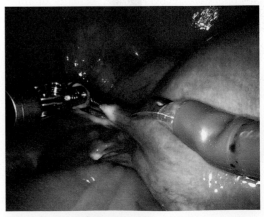

Fig. 4.2   Coagulating round ligament.

The posterior leaf of broad ligament is incised toward the uterosacral ligaments to skeletonize the uterine arteries. This step is done bilaterally, and ureters are identified.

- In case ovaries are to be removed, the infundibulopelvic ligaments are clamped, cauterized, and cut, but in cases where ovaries need to be preserved, utero ovarian ligaments are clamped, cauterized, and cut. The same procedure is repeated on contralateral side.
- Cervicovaginal junction is exposed by mobilizing the bladder off the cervix and upper vagina (**Fig. 4.3**).
- Uterine vessels are clamped, cauterized, and cut on both sides (**Fig. 4.4**).

- The cardinal ligaments are then clamped, cauterized, and transacted medially to the previous pedicle on both sides.
- The uterine manipulator should be pushed further inside to demarcate the colpotomy junction. Using monopolar scissors, colpotomy is done (**Fig. 4.5**), and the specimen is retrieved vaginally.
- Vault closure can be done using barbed sutures or Vicryl (**Fig. 4.6**).
- Hemostasis is rechecked and irrigation may be done if needed.
- Instruments are removed and dedocking of robot is done.
- Ports are removed under the vision and port closure stitches applied.

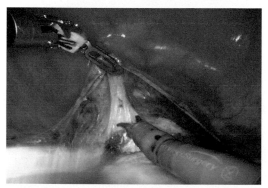

Fig. 4.3 Bladder pushed down.

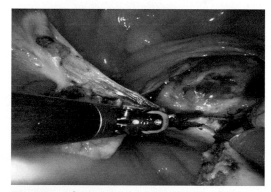

Fig. 4.4 Left uterine artery.

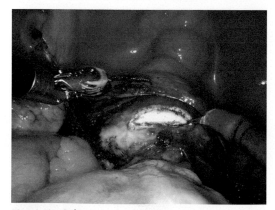

Fig. 4.5 Colpotomy incision.

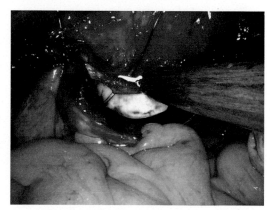

Fig. 4.6 Vault closure.

Postoperative Care

With the incorporation of enhanced recovery after surgery protocol, the patients can have free fluids on the day of surgery and breakfast on the following day itself.[8] Early catheter removal and ambulation enable the patient to get discharged within 24 to 48 hours. Abstinence is usually advised for 6 to 8 weeks postsurgery.

Complications

The main concerns during robotic surgery are a loss of tactile sensation resulting in poor handling of tissues and blunt surgical dissection.[9] According to the FDA database, operator-related errors and technical system failure account for 21% and 14%, respectively.[10] Lack of team communication, the intraoperative collision of surgical instruments, inadequate port and trocar placement, instruments going away from the camera view, and defects in protective sheaths of tools are other causes of robotic surgery complications.[11]

Risk of vaginal cuff dehiscence is higher in robotic approach (1.64%) as compared to 0.66% in laparoscopic group. Limiting the use of electrocautery during colpotomy, taking at least 5 mm of healthy vaginal tissue from the edge, providing better vault support by taking uterosacral ligaments, and avoiding vault trauma (avoiding intercourse and tampons for 6–12 weeks) are some measures to limit vaginal cuff dehiscence.[9]

No conflict of interest exists for this article.

No funding was needed for this article.

Acknowledgment

We sincerely thank Dr. Debashish, a third-year postgraduate student, for clicking the photographs.

References

1. Committee on Gynecologic. Committee Opinion No 701: choosing the route of hysterectomy for benign disease. Obstet Gynecol 2017;129(6):e155–e159
2. Aarts JW, Nieboer TE, Johnson N, et al. Surgical approach to hysterectomy for benign gynaecological disease. Cochrane Database Syst Rev 2015;8(8):CD003677
3. Nair R, Killicoat K, Ind TEJ. Robotic surgery in gynaecology. Obstet Gynaecol 2016;18: 221–229
4. O'Reilly BA. Patents running out: time to take stock of robotic surgery. Int Urogynecol J Pelvic Floor Dysfunct 2014;25(6):711–713
5. Diwadkar GB, Falcone T. Robotic surgery. In: Falcone T, Goldberg JM, eds. Basic, advanced and robotic laparoscopic surgery. Philadelphia, PA: Saunders (Elsevier); 2010:193–205
6. Diaz-Arrastia C, Jurnalov C, Gomez G, Townsend C Jr. Laparoscopic hysterectomy using a computer-enhanced surgical robot. Surg Endosc 2002;16(9):1271–1273
7. Gainsburg DM. Anesthetic concerns for robotic-assisted laparoscopic radical prostatectomy. Minerva Anestesiol 2012;78(5):596–604
8. Iavazzo C, Gkegkes ID. Enhanced recovery programme in robotic hysterectomy. Br J Nurs 2015;24(16):S4–S8
9. Tse KY, Ngan HYS, Lim PC. Robot-assisted gynaecological cancer surgery-complications and prevention. Best Pract Res Clin Obstet Gynaecol 2017;45:94–106
10. Manoucheri E, Fuchs-Weizman N, Cohen SL, Wang KC, Einarsson J. MAUDE: analysis of robotic-assisted gynecologic surgery. J Minim Invasive Gynecol 2014;21(4):592–595
11. Kohut A, Goldberg L, De Meritens AB. Robotic hysterectomy for cancer and benign pathology, new horizons in laparoscopic surgery, Murat Ferhat Ferhatoglu, IntechOpen. September 19, 2018. doi:10.5772/intechopen.76466. https://www.intechopen.com/books/new-horizons-in-laparoscopic-surgery/robotic-hysterectomy-for-cancer-and-benign-pathology

Accompanying Video

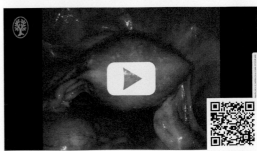

Video 4.1 Benign hysterectomy. https://www.thieme.de/de/q.htm?p=opn/cs/21/6/15245532-528352a8

5 Robotic Myomectomy

Anupama Bahadur, Divya Mishra, and Rajlaxmi Mundhra

Introduction

In the era of modern medicine, robot-assisted surgeries, commonly known as robotic surgeries, have carved a niche for themselves in the field of gynecologic surgeries. Since the approval of the da Vinci robotic system for gynecologic surgeries by U.S. FDA in 2005, robotic gynecologic procedures have been widely practiced and accepted by both surgeons and patients all over the world. It has evolved as an improvisation in continuum to the other form of minimally invasive surgery, (i.e., laparoscopy).

Compared to the six degrees of freedom of movement offered by human hands during a laparotomy, the robotic system provides an additional one, thus offering a total of seven degrees of freedom of instrument manipulation during surgery. This enables better dexterity and improves the efficiency, accuracy, and comfort associated with performing surgeries. In addition to the initial intent of using the da Vinci surgical system for performing robotic myomectomies and hysterectomies, it is also widely used for other benign and malignant conditions in gynecology tubal reanastomosis, complex endometriosis surgeries, and sacrocolpopexy.[1-3]

Robotic surgeries offer a broad spectrum of advantages over open as well as laparoscopic procedures. The most important among these include a three-dimensional visualization of the operating field, absence of tremor evidenced during manual handling of instruments, better articulation of instruments, and downscaling of movements. For the surgeon, it offers advantages of the comfort of operating and a faster learning curve as compared to the laparoscopic procedures.[4,5]

Robotic Myomectomy

Uterine leiomyomas are the most common benign tumors of the female reproductive tract. The gradually advancing age of child-bearing and modalities facilitating an early diagnosis of fibroids has led to an emerging need for uterine-sparing techniques in their surgical management. Traditionally, the removal of uterine fibroids has been taught by laparotomy, wherein the surgeon has the advantage of depth perception and feeling of tissue resistance for operative coordination. With the advent of laparoscopy, and further modification of laparoscopic operative techniques with electrosurgical devices and high-intensity light sources, the blood loss during myomectomies decreased. It also offered the benefit of lesser postoperative pain, shorter hospital stay, faster return to normal activities, and better cosmetic results. With the use of da Vinci robotic system, the dexterity of the surgeon improved. Tissue manipulation and dissection became easy and controlled. This was in addition to the seven degrees of freedom of instrumentation provided by the robotic system. There is another significant advantage offered by robotic myomectomy, in the form of ease of suturing with the help of robotic arms. This is beneficial for surgeons with limited laparoscopic experience, especially in endosuturing techniques. Not only is robotic myomectomy as meticulous as an open myomectomy, but it also is safe and acceptable, like laparoscopic myomectomy.[6]

In 2007, Advincula et al published their experience with robotic myomectomies in 35 patients with uterine leiomyomas.[7] The average number of fibroids removed during surgery in these patients was 1.6. The mean diameter of fibroids in their patients was 7.9 ± 3 cm with a mean fibroid weight of 223 ± 244 g. Their average operating time was reported to be 230 ± 83 minutes with a mean estimated blood loss of 169 ± 198 mL. The conversion rate from robotic to laparotomy was reported to be 8.6%, which is similar to that in laparoscopic myomectomy.

Subsequently, in 2013, Gobern et al reported their retrospective analysis of 66 robotic-assisted laparoscopic myomectomies.[8] The median size of myxomas removed robotically was 6.1 cm, with a median weight of 200 g. They drew comparisons with abdominal as well as laparoscopic myomectomies. They reported a median operating time of 140 minutes in robotic myomectomy, in contrast to a median of 70 minutes and 17 minutes for laparoscopic and abdominal myomectomies, respectively. The conversion rate to laparotomy was comparable between robotic and laparoscopic myomectomies in this study as well.

Indications, Patient Selection, and Preoperative Preparation

As robotic myomectomy is a relatively new surgery, variations in its technique exist among different centers. Appropriate patient selection for robotic myomectomy is an important initial step in surgical planning. The decision for appropriate route for surgical management of uterine fibroids should be taken after assessment of key anatomical factors like myopia size, extent, number, location, and proximity of the fibroid to uterine cavity. The surgeon's level of training and expertise, and the availability and affordability of surgical equipment, must be considered before choosing a surgical approach for myomectomy.

While deciding upon the approach for myomectomy, the suitable locations of fibroid for robotic surgery are subserosal, intramural, or fundal. A broad ligament or a pedunculated fibroid is generally considered ideal for robotic myomectomy.[9] Fibroids abutting the endometrial cavity, or fibroids with a submucosal component, may not be ideal for the robotic approach. These myomas pose a greater risk of entering the uterine cavity while operating, and closure of the cavity defect may be more complicated with the use of a robot due to lack of tactile feedback. Robotic myomectomy may not be considered appropriate in women with more than five myomas in the uterus or with a uterine size of more than 16 weeks. A robotic approach to myomectomy should be avoided if there is a single fibroid of size greater than 15 cm, or if the fibroid is located at anatomically challenging sites like near the cervix, uterine cornua, or uterine blood vessels. It should be noted that the decision for robotic myomectomy based on maximum size and number of uterine fibroids should be individualized, depending upon the surgeon's expertise and level of comfort. A preoperative magnetic resonance imaging (MRI) is advisable for all myomectomy candidates, not only to delineate the uterine dimensions and fibroid number, size, and exact location, but also to differentiate uterine fibroids from adenomyosis. The presence of diffuse myomatosis makes the patient a poor candidate for a robotic approach.

After the decision for robotic myomectomy has been taken, the preoperative preparation is similar to that in open or laparoscopic myomectomies. Preexisting anemia should be corrected, and in such patients, pretreatment with a GnRH-releasing hormone agonist should be considered to help reduce the fibroid and uterine volume.

Surgical Technique

The basic setup for robotic surgery consists of the patient side robot, a vision cart, and the robotic master console. Patient positioning and setup are similar to conventional laparoscopy. The patient is placed in dorsal lithotomy in Allen stirrups, with the arms padded and tucked on sides in neutral position. The robotic surgeon operates from the remote master console, with the help of hand controls and foot paddles. After the patient has been prepped and draped as for conventional gynecological laparoscopy, a uterine manipulator is inserted inside the uterus, and a Foley catheter is placed to drain the bladder.

The placement of trocars is decided based on the surgeon's preference. In general, a 12-mm infraumbilical optical trocar is used to enter the abdominal cavity. After performing a thorough survey of the abdominal and pelvic cavities and confirming that a robotic approach is appropriate, a robotic camera is placed through the same port. After this, two 8-mm robotic trocars are placed 8 to 12 cm lateral to the umbilical port

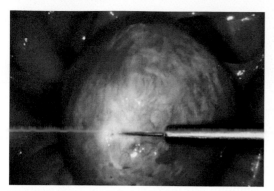

Fig. 5.1 Vasopressin being injected.

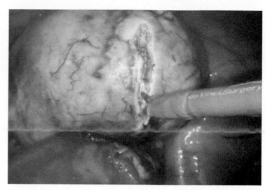

Fig. 5.2 Uterine incision.

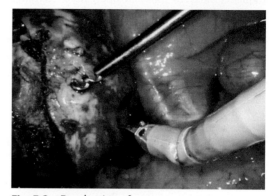

Fig. 5.3 Enucleation of myoma.

and at an angle of 15 degrees inferiorly. These two ports can be placed more cephalic in case of large uterine fibroids. Next, a 5-mm accessory port is placed in the left upper quadrant at the Palmers point, through which laparoscopic tenaculum forceps can be introduced for enucleation of fibroid. It can also be used for passing and handling needles.

After trocar placement, the patient is placed in Trendelenburg position, and the process of docking is completed. For this purpose, the robot with arms is placed either between the patient's legs or on the patient's side. Once the robotic arms are docked, the robotic camera and instruments are placed into their respective trocars. Usually, the preferred instruments are tenaculum forceps, Harmonic device, Maryland bipolar forceps connected to cautery, and needle drivers.

The fibroid position is confirmed by visual inspection and a dilute concentration of vasopressin is injected into the serosa and myometrium surrounding the fibroid, using a laparoscopic needle tip device (**Fig. 5.1**). The effectiveness of vasopressin, when injected into proper surgical planes, is demonstrated by blanching of the uterus. In the case of a pedunculated fibroid, vasopressin is injected directly into the fibroid stalk. Vasopressin should be used with caution owing to possible cardiovascular complications like bradycardia, hypertension, and cardiac arrest. It should be avoided in patients with hypertension and coronary artery disease. Other techniques used to decrease intraoperative blood loss include uterine artery ligation prior to myomectomy or temporary occlusion using catheters or elastic tourniquets.

After injecting vasopressin, an incision is made through the serosa and myometrium, deep enough to open the fibroid capsule (**Fig. 5.2**). Every attempt should be made to make the incision away from the fallopian tubes, ovaries, cornua, and uterine vessels. Traditionally, the incision was made transversely for the ease of suturing. Now, with the robotic equipment, incision and suturing can be done vertically also. Hemostasis during surgery can be achieved using electrocautery or thrombin-infused gelatin products. After entering the myoma capsule and exposing the myoma fibers, the fibroid is held using tenaculum forceps or myoma screw and is enucleated using blunt dissection and traction, along with harmonic energy as required (**Fig. 5.3**). Excessive traction on the myoma should be avoided to prevent the opening of the endometrial cavity, especially when the desired outcome of myomectomy is the preservation of fertility. Chromopertubation with methylene blue dye can be done to check for endometrial integrity. Pedunculated fibroids are removed by transecting their stalk using a ligature device. While removing broad ligament fibroids, the utmost caution should be practiced to avoid injury to the ureters and surrounding uterine blood vessels. The removed fibroids are placed in the rectouterine pouch or the paracolic gutters. The surgical team must count the total number of enucleated myomas to avoid leaving any myoma behind during specimen retrieval and morcellation.

The next step is the multilayer closure of the uterine incision, using sutures and suturing techniques similar to those in open myomectomy. For this purpose, barbed sutures are preferred, as they do not require a knot, and the tension is distributed along the entire length of the suture, without the need for applying constant pressure while suturing. Robotic surgery offers the benefit of ease and speed of suturing, limiting the intraoperative blood loss. This is further aided by the use of barbed sutures.[10] Adequate myometrial closure and obliteration of dead space are essential issues while translating open surgical techniques to robotic surgery. The closure of uterine serosa is accomplished using the baseball-stitch method. An adhesion barrier may be placed onto the closed hysterotomy to prevent future scar tissue formation.

The power morcellator was commonly used in the past for removal of enucleated myomas at the end of surgery. However, the concerns regarding the potential risk of spreading an occult uterine leiomyosarcoma have led to the practice of its limited use. The American Association of Gynecologic Laparoscopists (AAGL) highlights that there is not enough data at this time to recommend against power morcellation in properly selected patients, who are at low risk for the presence of uterine or cervical malignancy or premalignant conditions.

After the removal of all the fibroids, the robot can be undocked. All of the robotic arms are unlocked from respective trocars, and the robot is pulled away from the patient. The trocars are then removed under direct visualization and the fascia underlying the umbilical port is closed, followed by skin closure.

Postoperative Care

The postoperative care after a robotic myomectomy is similar to that after a laparoscopic myomectomy, with the essential goals being early mobilization, pain control, and early discharge from the hospital. Depending upon the extent of surgical procedure, disruption of the uterine myometrium, and entry into the uterine endometrium, the patient should be counseled regarding the possible need for a cesarean section and the increased risk of uterine rupture in the future. The operative notes and recommendations must be documented by the surgeon for the purpose of planning of mode of delivery in the future.

Surgical Outcomes, Advantages, and Limitations

The most significant advantage of robotic myomectomy is that it offers the surgeon the ability to apply open surgical techniques in a minimally invasive fashion, thus providing the opportunity of performing a minimally invasive surgery for myomectomy in patients who would have otherwise required a traditional laparotomy for removal of their fibroid. Robotic myomectomy is generally a safe procedure, and provides a valid alternative to open myomectomy for appropriately selected surgical patients. It is associated with a lesser operative blood loss, shorter hospital stay, better cosmesis and analgesia, rapid return of bowel function, and faster return to normal activities. It can be performed safely in patients with high body mass index, and obesity does not necessarily affect the surgical outcomes. In contrast to conventional laparoscopy, robotic myomectomy can be performed without positioning the patient in a steep Trendelenburg position, thus making it suitable for those patients who cannot safely sustain such a position.

The robot provides a three-dimensional image of the operating field, facilitating improved and precise suture handling and ease of suturing. The robotic endoscopic instruments mimic the dexterity of human hands and provide a greater range of motion and depth perception to increase surgical precision. They also facilitate motion scaling, thus eliminating tremors. In contrast to traditional laparoscopy, the da Vinci robotic system gives autonomous control over the camera and the instruments, thereby reducing surgical fatigue. The enhanced dexterity enables the surgeon to do more gentle tissue handling and dissection, which favors future reproductive outcomes and results in high pregnancy rates in patients who have undergone robotic myomectomy.

The significant limitations of da Vinci robotic system are the increased cost of its establishment, the need for personnel training, and an extended operating time. The surgeons performing robotic procedures report a decrease in the operating time with increasing experience with the robotic system. Another disadvantage is the lack of tactile feedback during robotic procedures, which may lead to suture breakage or application of excessive traction on the myoma, resulting in breach in the endometrial cavity. The robotic ports are slightly larger than those in conventional laparoscopy and are placed a little higher in the abdominal cavity. This makes the conversion to laparotomy more challenging, if required, compared to traditional laparoscopy. The robotic system is space occupying, and any position changing requires undocking and redocking the robot, increasing the operating time and resultant cost-effectiveness of the procedure.

Like with other methods of myomectomy, robotic myomectomy also poses a future risk of recurrence of the myomas. There is still insufficient data pertaining to the long-term quality of life and obstetric outcomes following a robotic myomectomy. More studies are required to ascertain these outcomes in the future.

References

1. Chen CC, Falcone T. Robotic gynecologic surgery: past, present, and future. Clin Obstet Gynecol 2009;52(3):335–343
2. Magrina JF. Robotic surgery in gynecology. Eur J Gynaecol Oncol 2007;28(2):77–82
3. Holloway RW, Patel SD, Ahmad S. Robotic surgery in gynecology. Scand J Surg 2009; 98(2):96–109
4. Quaas AM, Einarsson JI, Srouji S, Gargiulo AR. Robotic myomectomy: a review of indications and techniques. Rev Obstet Gynecol 2010; 3(4):185–191
5. Truong M, Kim JH, Scheib S, Patzkowsky K. Advantages of robotics in benign gynecologic surgery. Curr Opin Obstet Gynecol 2016; 28(4):304–310
6. Sinha R, Sanjay M, Rupa B, Kumari S. Robotic surgery in gynecology. J Minim Access Surg 2015;11(1):50–59
7. Advincula AP, Xu X, Goudeau S IV, Ransom SB. Robot-assisted laparoscopic myomectomy versus abdominal myomectomy: a comparison of short-term surgical outcomes and immediate costs. J Minim Invasive Gynecol 2007; 14(6):698–705
8. Gobern JM, Rosemeyer CJ, Barter JF, Steren AJ. Comparison of robotic, laparoscopic, and abdominal myomectomy in a community hospital. JSLS 2013;17(1):116–120
9. Seracchioli R, Rossi S, Govoni F, et al. Fertility and obstetric outcome after laparoscopic myomectomy of large myomata: a randomized comparison with abdominal myomectomy. Hum Reprod 2000;15(12):2663–2668
10. Einarsson JI, Chavan NR, Suzuki Y, Jonsdottir G, Vellinga TT, Greenberg JA. Use of bidirectional barbed suture in laparoscopic myomectomy: evaluation of perioperative outcomes, safety, and efficacy. J Minim Invasive Gynecol 2011; 18(1):92–95

6 Robotic Sacrocolpopexy

Farhanul Huda and Praveen Kumar

Introduction

Aging women commonly encounter pelvic organ prolapse (POP) and associated urinary, bowel, and sexual dysfunction. According to an estimate, one in nine women undergo surgery for POP till they reach 80 years.[1] Treatment options can be surgical or nonsurgical. POP is defined as the descent of the anterior, posterior, and/or apical vaginal compartments with protrusion of one or more pelvic organs (e.g., bladder, uterus, posthysterectomy vaginal cuff, small bowel, or rectum) into the vagina.[2] Loss of structural support leads to pathologic changes that alter the quality of life of a woman.

Anatomical Supports

Pelvic floor support is made up of dynamic interactions between muscles and connective tissue attachments within the bony pelvis. Muscular support is provided by levator ani muscles, which form the pelvic diaphragm. There are three components of the levator ani, namely, pubococcygeus, iliococcygeus, and puborectalis. These muscles are attached to the true pelvis inner surface to form the muscular floor.[3] Coccygeus muscle is also involved in pelvic support; it arises from the ischial spine and is inserted into coccyx and lower sacrum. Fascial supports are provided by arcus tendinous levator ani, urogenital diaphragm, perineal body, and cardinal and uterosacral ligaments complex. There are three levels of vaginal connective tissue support of the pelvis: Level I is at the apex of the vagina and is by the cardinal and uterosacral ligament complex, which suspends the vagina by attaching it to pelvic sidewalls. Level II is by arcus tendinous fascia pelvis which gives support to the lateral walls of the vagina. Level III support is the most distal where the vagina fuses with the urogenital diaphragm. Loss of apical vaginal support most commonly leads to POP; it can be associated with loss of support along the lateral vaginal wall. The apical compartment includes the uterus, cervix, or vaginal cuff after hysterectomy. In POP, restoration of apical support is most important and helps prevent failures in other compartments.[4,5]

Pathophysiology

Advancing age is associated with POP due to physiologic changes in pelvic floor components and decline in estrogen during the postmenopausal period. Estrogen influences the synthesis and degradation of collagen, which is the main constituent of connective tissue of the pelvis. Estrogen increases muscle and connective strength of the pelvis by increasing collagen type I expression and overall cross-link concentration of collagen. Type I collagen is found in organized fibers and ligaments, which provides strong structural support, whereas type III collagen is found in loose areolar tissue, which provides weak structural support. Estrogen increases pelvic support by increasing type I collagen and decreasing type III collagen.[6] It decreases degradation of collagen and elastin by reducing matrix metalloproteinases (MMPs), a family of zinc-dependent endopeptidases responsible for degradation of collagen and by increasing cystatin C which promotes crosslinking of collagen by inhibiting cathepsin.[7] Pregnancy and childbirth induce physiologic changes in pelvic floor musculature and connective tissue for preparing the pelvic floor for vaginal birth. High levels of progesterone during pregnancy cause smooth muscle relaxation and antagonize the effects of estrogen. Chronically raised intra-abdominal pressure due to chronic constipation, high BMI, chronic cough, and repetitive weight lifting also play a role in pathogenesis. History of hysterectomy and loss of any level of support like apical, midvaginal, and distal also lead to prolapse.

Clinical Features and Staging

The most common symptom of POP is a vaginal bulge, which occurs in 94 to 100% of cases[8]; other symptoms like pelvic pain or pressure, urgency, incontinence, frequency, back pain, bowel symptoms, and dyspareunia are present in varying frequencies. POP is staged using Baden-Walker or POP-quantification (POP-Q) classification[9]:

- Stage 0: No prolapse.
- Stage I: Distal prolapse >1 cm proximal to the hymen.
- Stage II: Distal prolapse within 1 cm of hymen, either proximal or distal.
- Stage III: Distal prolapse >1 cm below hymen without complete eversion.
- Stage IV: Complete vaginal eversion.

Diagnostic Workup

Detailed history, including psychosomatic questions, examination for prolapse in all compartments like anterior, apical, and posterior, and ruling out occult stress incontinence by the clinical stress test, is critical in planning appropriate surgical procedures and any concomitant surgical procedure if required. The patient should be asked to maintain a micturition diary. Basic tests include urinalysis to rule out infection and postvoid residual urine by ultrasonography. Perineal or introital ultrasound will determine bladder neck mobility or funneling. To evaluate micturition, uroflowmetry, and to know the filling behavior of the bladder, a urodynamic study should be done. Cystoscopy should also be done, which usually shows chronic changes in the bladder. Dynamic magnetic resonance (MR) defecography is used for morphologic and functional evaluation of all three compartments simultaneously, enabling real-time assessment of morphologic and functional diseases.[10]

Treatment Options

Active treatment is indicated if symptoms are bothersome to the patient. Patients who wish to avoid surgery can be treated with a pessary.[11] Surgical options include obliterative and restorative procedures. Colpocleisis is the obliterative procedure and is reserved for those patients who do not want to preserve their sexual function. Restorative procedures include transvaginal primary repair with or without mesh, abdominal sacrocolpopexy (ASC), laparoscopic sacrocolpopexy (LSC), and robotic sacrocolpopexy (RSC).

ASC has been the gold standard for apical support defect with a roughly 75% anatomical success rate at 7 years and has surpassed vaginal repairs, a 60 to 70% failure rate at 5 years. LSC is considered superior to ASC due to shorter recovery time, reduced pain, and shorter hospital stay.[12] A longitudinal 7-year study on LSC on 280 women has reported only a 3.3% repeat surgery rate for recurrent POP.[13] However, LSC is technically challenging due to suture intensive nature, dissection around common iliac vessels, longer learning curve; all these have limited its widespread use. These problems are overcome by the use of robotics in sacrocolpopexy; its improved vision and ergonomics by wristed movements have allowed more surgeons to adopt RSC. Although meta-analysis has demonstrated similar outcomes of RSC over LSC, its technical feasibility in terms of three-dimensional view, increased degrees of freedom in movement, and easy knot tying have made RSC a favorite among surgeons.[14] The first study on RSC of five patients was published by Di Marco et al in 2004,[15] since then more and more surgeons have shifted toward RSC for POP.

Technique of Robotic Sacrocolpopexy

Basic Setup

It consists of a vision cart, a master console, and a patient-side robot. The original da Vinci system had three arms, two operative arms, and one camera arm; the addition of extra arm to the existing system allows retraction and better exposure and freedom to have better control during all aspects of the procedure. At the console, the surgeon controls the robot by hand controls and foot pedals. The operative arms of robot are guided by finger grip handle that moves up and down, left and right, in and out. The clutch foot pedal helps the surgeon change control from operative arms to the camera or third instrument arm. Separate foot pedal controls instrument for cauterization. The camera has a unique binocular vision for three-dimensional image on master console. Despite the surgeon on the master console controlling the robot, a bedside assistant must provide additional retraction, suction, and exchange of instruments.

Patient Positioning

Robotic surgery requires specific positioning of the patient, while open sacrocolpopexy uses a low lithotomy position to allow access to the lower abdomen and vagina simultaneously. RSC uses steep Trendelenburg (>45 degrees) for adequate access for robotic arms to pelvis without interference. Positioning requires proper stabilization of the upper body to prevent sliding of the patient. The robot is positioned at the foot end of the bed between the legs of the patient. Sometimes side docking may be required for easy access to the vagina for manipulation by the assistant.

Port Placements

Ports are placed in a pyramidal or triangular configuration. A 12-mm camera port is placed at or near the umbilicus. First port placement is by open or closed technique, followed by CO_2 insufflation. 8-mm robotic ports are placed at the rectus muscle's lateral edge, thus preventing injury to epigastric vessels.[9] The fourth arm of the robot is placed laterally, usually above the left anterior superior iliac spine. The assistant port is 10 to 12 mm, the position is variable, and sometimes an additional 5-mm port may be required. A total of five to six ports are placed and the distance between ports should be approximately 9 cm to avoid the collision.

Surgical Technique

Adhesiolysis

After placing all ports, adhesions are lysed with standard laparoscopy. Small bowel is brought into the abdominal cavity from the pelvis with the help of a bowel grasper once the patient is placed in steep Trendelenburg position. The sigmoid colon is retracted and mobilized using the fourth robotic arm. Clamping of the colon with a robotic arm need not be done to avoid colonic perforation. Some surgeons prefer a percutaneous suture be passed through the colonic serosa and clamped at the skin for retraction.[15,16]

Identification of Sacral Promontory

Next step is to identify sacral promontory by following pelvic brim to the base of the sigmoid mesentery medially and the pulsatile iliac artery laterally. The right ureter can be used as useful landmark, and is identified through the peritoneum with its characteristic peristalsis. Another useful method of identifying the promontory is that the ureter is present approximately 30 mm lateral to sacral promontory, so measuring 30 mm medial to ureter along pelvic brim is the most likely position of sacral promontory.[17] After identifying the promontory, peritoneum is lifted off bony promontory and opened with monopolar cautery, to continue dissection until anterior longitudinal ligament is identified. Visible prominent vessels should be controlled with bipolar cautery. Middle sacral artery should be avoided. After identification of ligament, peritoneum is incised caudally and medially to the vaginal apex, creating a gutter where the mesh is placed as an interposition between the vagina and sacral promontory.

Vaginal Dissection

Vaginal dissection is an essential step of the procedure; vaginal manipulation by bedside assistant with sponge stick is necessary for robotic dissection. Elliott et al described vaginal manipulation by specialized instrument with a long handle at the right angle for easy manipulation by an assistant, with the robot being docked at the foot end of bed.[18] Plane of dissection between bladder and vagina is bloodless; any bleeding alarms entry into bladder detrusor muscle or vaginal muscularis. Preoperative Foley catheter placement and retrograde filling of the bladder aid in identifying the bladder margins. The extent of anterior dissection has been an issue, but now the generally accepted rule is to reach as close as possible to trigone to prevent a recurrence but avoid dissecting deep to the trigone. According to a recent publication, measuring the bladder neck-mesh distance (BMD) using transvaginal ultrasound is useful. A BMD of greater than 6 mm is ideal for preventing postoperative symptoms.[19] The surgeon should dissect sufficiently to detach anterior and posterior vaginal walls to fix the mesh arms appropriately; approximately upper one-third of vagina, and posterior vaginal wall should be dissected from the rectum to reach rectovaginal space.

Mesh Placement

Pore size is more important than the chemical composition of mesh. Macroporous mesh is better as it allows macrophages and leukocytes to enter and prevent infection. Macroporous and mono-filament [Type I] polypropylene mesh should be used.[20] A Y-shaped polypropylene mesh is most commonly used. Y-shaped mesh fixes anterior and posterior vaginal walls to sacral promontory, with nonabsorbable suture like PTFE (Gore-Tex), as this material is easier to tie and there are fewer chances of breakage. A recent randomized study by Tan-Kim et al found no significant difference between anatomic failure rate at 12 months postoperative with the use of continuous barbed suture and interrupted nonbarbed sutures for anchoring the mesh to the vaginal wall.[21] A follow-up study reported that delayed-absorption barbed suture to fix the mesh to the vaginal wall had no recurrence or mesh exposure.[22] Another important consideration is the fixation of the mesh at the sacral promontory. The most prominent point of the sacral promontory is the L5–S1 disk which is easy to locate during surgery, but penetration of the disk during fixation leads to diskitis. To prevent this, the mesh can be fixed to the body of S1 which is located 5 mm inferior to the most prominent point of promontory.[23] If the surgeon is not sure of S1 body, avoid a deep bite, not more than 1 to 2 mm thick, which is the thickness of anterior

longitudinal ligament, to prevent postoperative diskitis. After mesh fixation, the peritoneum should be closed to avoid bowel adhesions.

Concomitant Procedure

Hysterectomy is the most common procedure performed with RSC in those women who do not want to preserve their childbearing function. RSC with concomitant hysterectomy is associated with low complication rates compared to sacrocolpopexy alone.[24] RSC and total hysterectomy are associated with high rates of mesh exposure[25] but lower rates of recurrent anterior vaginal prolapse in contrast to supracervical hysterectomy. In women of childbearing age or who wish to preserve their uterus, sacrohysteropexy can be performed.

Anti-incontinence procedures are the subsequent most common procedures with RSC. It is challenging to decide which patients will need an anti-incontinence procedure. Brubaker et al described prophylactic Bursch procedures with ASC and improvement in stress urinary incontinence in CARE trial, regardless of the fact that whether the patient had preoperative SUI or not.[26] No such data is available with RSC, but midurethral slings are performed with RSC most commonly in up to 70% of cases.[27]

Complications

Sacrocolpopexy is associated with ureteric injury, vascular or bowel injury at the time of trocar insertion, epigastric vessel injury, port site hernia, mesh exposure, bladder injury, and complications of sacral component like a hemorrhage from presacral vessels and diskitis. RSC has its own set of complications; steep Trendelenburg position can lead to difficult ventilation in morbidly obese and those with underlying lung pathology. Technical failure of the robot can happen; conversion to laparoscopy or open procedure is desired. According to systematic reviews conducted by Serati et al and Hudson et al, the conversion rate of RSC to open surgery was 0 to 8.6%, and overall complication rate was 10%. According to Clavin-Dindo classification, all complications were from Grade 1 to Grade 3b; no complication was Grade 4 to Grade 5. Mesh erosion rate is relatively low with ASC, which is

0–8% with RSC. The use of robotic per se does not increase the chances of mesh erosion.[28,29]

Efficacy and Safety of Robotic Sacrocolpopexy

Open sacrocolpopexy has been considered as a suitable procedure for apical prolapse, with success rate of 78 to 100%, but it is associated with the increased analgesic requirement, length of stay, and increased cost when compared with transvaginal procedures.[30] LSC and RSC have overall decreased morbidity and good anatomical success as compared to ASC.[31] LSC has overcome many limitations of ASC, but LSC is more technically demanding and has a steep learning curve. Since 2004, with the adoption of RSC, surgeons have become more comfortable with the procedure with good dexterity, without many technical demands and a learning curve. A systematic review conducted in 2014 by Serati et al showed an apical cure rate of 97 to 100%, and overall cure rate in all compartments was 84 to 100%. Relapse was present in 6.4% of patients, and 3.4%, 0.4%, and 2.6%, respectively, in anterior, apical, and posterior compartments. Reoperation rate was 3.3%, out of which 0.4% was for apical and rest for nonapical compartments.[28] Van Zanten et al conducted a prospective observational study on 144 patients with follow-up of at least 1 year, which reported that cure rate of apical prolapse was 91% after 12 months, the overall cure rate was 67%, and the recurrence rate was 20.9% in all compartments with a minimum of 0.7% in apical compartment.[24] In another systematic review conducted by Hudson et al in 2014, the anatomic cure rate was 98.6% for RSC with a mean follow-up of 26.9 months.[29]

Estimated blood loss in RSC was 50 to 82.5 mL, hospital stay was 2 to 2.4 days, and median surgery time was 194 minutes with a range of 75 to 536 minutes. A wide range was due to concurrent procedures.[28,29]

Recently the cure rate shifted toward subjective cure rate, which includes improvement in overall symptoms and patient's satisfaction with the outcome; it does not meet strict anatomic success measured by POP-Q stages. Parameters evaluated are symptom improvement utilizing validated questionnaires. The subjective cure

rate with RSC is 95%, and the satisfaction rate is 95 to 100%.[24,28]

Limitations

The most critical limitation is cost, including purchasing the system, annual maintenance costs, and the cost of robotic instruments, which have a life for a limited number of cases.

Recent Advances in RSC

After seeing mesh-related complications like mesh erosion in 0-8% of patients,[24,28] meshless options are evaluated. Native tissue procedures like uterosacral ligament suspension have been performed recently with good outcomes.[32] Long-term trials are needed to establish the efficacy of such practices.

The single-port approach is being adopted in minimal access surgery with good cosmesis and decreased morbidity. Reports on single-port RSC are available, and it is being accepted.[33]

The sacral component of the procedure is associated with complications like bleeding, diskitis, and ureteral injury. To avoid all these complications, Banerjee and Noe in 2011 described pectopexy, which involves the suspension of vaginal apex using two mesh arms to the lateral ileopectineal ligaments as opposed to sacral promontory.[34]

Conclusion

Sacrocolpopexy is the procedure of choice for apical prolapse for women willing to preserve their sexual function. Minimal access techniques offer similar outcomes with fewer side effects. After the introduction of robotic surgery, this technique has taken over as it is technically less demanding. Newer techniques like single-port, pectopexy, and meshless techniques have further reduced complications. Long-term evaluation of outcomes of this technique is needed. With newer and improved robotic platforms and efforts to bring down the costs, the future of robotics is bright.

References

1. Olsen AL, Smith VJ, Bergstrom JO, Colling JC, Clark AL. Epidemiology of surgically managed pelvic organ prolapse and urinary incontinence. Obstet Gynecol 1997;89(4):501–506
2. DeLancey JO. The hidden epidemic of pelvic floor dysfunction: achievable goals for improved prevention and treatment. Am J Obstet Gynecol 2005;192(5):1488–1495
3. Maldonado PA, Wai CY. Pelvic organ prolapse: new concepts in pelvic floor anatomy. Obstet Gynecol Clin North Am 2016;43(1):15–26
4. Brubaker L, Maher C, Jacquetin B, Rajamaheswari N, von Theobald P, Norton P. Surgery for pelvic organ prolapse. Female Pelvic Med Reconstr Surg 2010;16(1):9–19
5. Hsu Y, Chen L, Summers A, Ashton-Miller JA, DeLancey JO. Anterior vaginal wall length and degree of anterior compartment prolapse seen on dynamic MRI. Int Urogynecol J Pelvic Floor Dysfunct 2008;19(1):137–142
6. Clark AL, Slayden OD, Hettrich K, Brenner RM. Estrogen increases collagen I and III mRNA expression in the pelvic support tissues of the rhesus macaque. Am J Obstet Gynecol 2005;192(5):1523–1529
7. Zhou L, Shangguan AJ, Kujawa SA, et al. Estrogen and pelvic organ prolapse. J Mol Genet Med 2016;10:221. ISSN 1747–0862
8. DeLancey JO. Anatomic aspects of vaginal eversion after hysterectomy. Am J Obstet Gynecol 1992;166(6 Pt 1):1717–1724, discussion 1724–1728
9. Kaboshi K. Evaluation of patients with urinary incontinence and pelvic organ prolapse. In: Wein AJ, Kavoussi LR, Novick AC, Partin AW, Peters CA, eds. Campbell Walsh urology. 10th ed. Philadelphia, PA: WB Saunders; 2012: 1896–908
10. Maccioni F. Functional disorders of the ano-rectal compartment of the pelvic floor: clinical and diagnostic value of dynamic MRI. Abdom Imaging 2013;38(5):930–951
11. Lamers BH, Broekman BM, Milani AL. Pessary treatment for pelvic organ prolapse and health-related quality of life: a review. Int Urogynecol J Pelvic Floor Dysfunct 2011;22(6):637–644
12. Nygaard I, Brubaker L, Zyczynski HM, et al. Long-term outcomes following abdominal sacrocolpopexy for pelvic organ prolapse. JAMA 2013;309(19):2016–2024
13. Pacquée S, Nawapun K, Claerhout F, et al. Long-term assessment of a prospective cohort of patients undergoing laparoscopic sacrocolpopexy. Obstet Gynecol 2019;134(2): 323–332
14. Liu H, Lawrie TA, Lu D, Song H, Wang L, Shi G. Robot-assisted surgery in gynaecology. Cochrane Database Syst Rev 2014;(12): CD011422
15. Di Marco DS, Chow GK, Gettman MT, Elliott DS. Robotic-assisted laparoscopic sacrocolpopexy for treatment of vaginal vault prolapse. Urology 2004;63(2):373–376
16. Akl MN, Long JB, Giles DL, et al. Robotic-assisted sacrocolpopexy: technique and learning curve. Surg Endosc 2009;23(10):2390–2394
17. McCullough M, Valceus J, Downes K, Hoyte L. The ureter as a landmark for robotic sacro-colpopexy. Female Pelvic Med Reconstr Surg 2012;18(3):162–164
18. Elliott DS, Krambeck AE, Chow GK. Long-term results of robotic assisted laparoscopic sacrocolpopexy for the treatment of high grade vaginal vault prolapse. J Urol 2006;176(2):655–659
19. Habib N, Centini G, Pizzoferrato AC, Bui C, Argay I, Bader G. Laparoscopic promontofixation: where to stop the anterior dissection? Med Hypotheses 2019;124:60–63
20. Warembourg S, Labaki M, de Tayrac R, Costa P, Fatton B. Reoperations for mesh-related complications after pelvic organ prolapse repair: 8-year experience at a tertiary referral center. Int Urogynecol J Pelvic Floor Dysfunct 2017;28(8):1139–1151
21. Tan-Kim J, Nager CW, Grimes CL, et al. A randomized trial of vaginal mesh attachment techniques for minimally invasive sacrocolpopexy. Int Urogynecol J Pelvic Floor Dysfunct 2015;26(5):649–656
22. Borahay MA, Oge T, Walsh TM, Patel PR, Rodriguez AM, Kilic GS. Outcomes of robotic sacrocolpopexy using barbed delayed absorbable sutures. J Minim Invasive Gynecol 2014; 21(3):412–416
23. Abernethy M, Vasquez E, Kenton K, Brubaker L, Mueller E. Where do we place the sacro-colpopexy stitch? A magnetic resonance imaging investigation. Female Pelvic Med Reconstr Surg 2013;19(1):31–33
24. van Zanten F, Schraffordt Koops SE, O'Sullivan OE, Lenters E, Broeders I, O'Reilly BA. Robot-assisted surgery for the management of apical prolapse: a bi-centre prospective cohort study. BJOG 2019;126(8):1065–1073

25. Osmundsen BC, Clark A, Goldsmith C, et al. Mesh erosion in robotic sacrocolpopexy. Female Pelvic Med Reconstr Surg 2012;18(2):86–88

26. Brubaker L, Nygaard I, Richter HE, et al. Two-year outcomes after sacrocolpopexy with and without burch to prevent stress urinary incontinence. Obstet Gynecol 2008;112(1): 49–55

27. Salamon CG, Lewis C, Priestley J, Gurshumov E, Culligan PJ. Prospective study of an ultra-lightweight polypropylene Y mesh for robotic sacrocolpopexy. Int Urogynecol J Pelvic Floor Dysfunct 2013;24(8):1371–1375

28. Serati M, Bogani G, Sorice P, et al. Robot-assisted sacrocolpopexy for pelvic organ prolapse: a systematic review and meta-analysis of comparative studies. Eur Urol 2014;66(2):303–318

29. Hudson CO, Northington GM, Lyles RH, Karp DR. Outcomes of robotic sacrocolpopexy: a systematic review and meta-analysis. Female Pelvic Med Reconstr Surg 2014;20(5):252–260

30. Lee RK, Mottrie A, Payne CK, Waltregny D. A review of the current status of laparoscopic and robot-assisted sacrocolpopexy for pelvic organ prolapse. Eur Urol 2014;65(6):1128–1137

31. Nosti PA, Umoh Andy U, Kane S, et al. Outcomes of abdominal and minimally invasive sacrocolpopexy: a retrospective cohort study. Female Pelvic Med Reconstr Surg 2014; 20(1):33–37

32. Davila HH, Gallo T, Bruce L, Landrey C. Robotic and laparoendoscopic single-site utero-sacral ligament suspension for apical vaginal prolapse: evaluation of our technique and perioperative outcomes. J Robot Surg 2017;11(2): 171–177

33. Guan X, Ma Y, Gisseman J, Kleithermes C, Liu J. Robotic single-site sacrocolpopexy using barbed suture anchoring and peritoneal tunneling technique: tips and tricks. J Minim Invasive Gynecol 2017;24(1):12–13

34. Banerjee C, Noé KG. Laparoscopic pectopexy: a new technique of prolapse surgery for obese patients. Arch Gynecol Obstet 2011; 284(3):631–635

7 Role of Robotic Surgery in Pelvic Endometriosis

Anshumala Shukla Kulkarni and Shweta Shetye

Endometriosis is a gynecologic disorder defined as the presence of endometrial glands and stroma outside the uterine cavity. It affects an estimated 6 to 15% of reproductive-age women,[1] 20 to 50% of infertile women,[2] and 71 to 87% of women with chronic pelvic pain.[3] Worldwide, there are over 70 million women and adolescents affected by endometriosis with an estimated 5.5 million women in the United States and Canada, and approximately 51,000 hospitalizations for endometriosis yearly. The disease results in decreased quality of life, ranging from chronic pelvic pain to infertility.[4] The range of severity of the disease can vary widely, as can the means of treating it.[5,6] Current recommendations include treatment with a trial of nonsteroidal anti-inflammatory agents and hormonal therapy, such as progesterone, oral contraceptives, aromatase inhibitors, or gonadotropin-releasing hormone agonists, but eradication by surgical means is often the most effective treatment.[7] Depending on the pervasiveness of the disease, multiple surgical interventions may be indicated to manage this condition successfully.

Surgical interventions have moved from open laparotomy to increased use of minimal invasive surgery to treat the disease.[7] The complexity of the disease can range from a grade 1 minimal involvement to grade 4 endometriosis, which has all organs in the pelvis involved. Traditional laparoscopy scored over open surgery due to less pain, reduced hospital stay, reduced complications, the magnified view of the telescope, and the capability of reaching into the pouch of Douglas and visualizing the smaller lesions.[8–10] The technique of surgical management of endometriosis has changed from ablation alone with use of bipolar current, which was ineffective in cases of deep infiltrative endometriosis, to excisional surgery for endometriosis. Excisional endometriosis surgery involves extensive dissection and removal of all endometriotic implants. In severe form of endometriosis, the most common involvement is seen at the uterosacral and ureters and the rectosigmoid.

The limitation of traditional laparoscopy, loss of depth perception in two-dimensional vision, and straight stick instruments with counterintuitive movement, operator fatigue, tremors, and lack of proper instrumentation impedes the use of laparoscopy to treat endometriosis by an average surgeon.[11–13] Robotic technology has managed to bridge the gap between open surgery and laparoscopic surgery.

The enhanced vision of the immersive 3D high-definition view helps in precision while performing adhesiolysis.[14–17] Endometriosis is seen with grades of adhesions of ovaries with pelvic side wall, adherent rectum to either uterosacral or pouch of Douglas, ureters adherent to ovarian cysts. The precision of dissection is the key to prevention of injuries to these organs.

The Xi generation of the da Vinci robot has inbuilt green filter which is used to identify indocyanine green (ICG) dye in lymph nodes or in any vascular channel. Endometriosis is a highly vascular disease; the ectopic endometrial implants are capable of neoangiogenesis and self-proliferation. Endometriosis lesions can be challenging to identify in the atypical forms such as vesicular lesions, white lesions, and peritoneal pockets. In the pelvis, the depth of the lesion can be as deep as 2 cm, and excision of the entire lesion is necessary for pain relief. The role of ICG dye here is to identify these vascular deposits and delineate the depth of the nodule to help complete excision.

The robotic system allows wristed movements; the appropriate use of these movements is in the dissection into the pelvic cavity. In case of a frozen pelvis where the uterus is buried between the bladder and the rectal adhesions and ovaries are adherent posteriorly, the approach to hysterectomy is only laterally; this involves opening the space lateral to the ureters or the Latzko space. Lateral identification of the ureter is the first step, following which the IP is ligated, and the medial pararectal space or the Okabayashi space is opened to help rectal dissection (**Figs. 7.1** to **7.4**). Experts at laparoscopy also find the approach difficult and requiring multiple points of traction-countertraction, which means multiple ports. The extra robotic arm increases the surgeon's control on traction, and the access achieved with the camera and wristed instruments helps to dissect and unfreeze the frozen pelvis. Ureteroneocystostomy, a procedure done when there is ureteric obstruction with endometriosis growing over or inside the ureter, requires dissection, and precision of suture anastomosis; robotic instruments with fine needle holders can use finer sutures to achieve this.

The robotic approach is often criticized for not having haptics, hence not allowing the feel of the tissue and nodule. The improved vision and dissection make haptics of less value and use of ICG dye helps.

Research and observational studies conducted on robotic surgery for endometriosis have shown merit in obese patients and those requiring extensive surgery.

A recent retrospective cohort study by Nezhat et al[18] compared laparoscopic versus robotic surgery performed by a single surgeon at the center. They compared all patients with stage III or stage IV endometriosis having surgery by both techniques for extent of surgery, estimated blood loss, operating room time, intraoperative and postoperative complications, and length of stay. Results showed higher body mass index (BMI) patients underwent robotic surgery though they required longer operative time.

Scant published data exist comparing the robotic minimally invasive approach with the conventional laparoscopic approach for the treatment of endometriosis. A retrospective study by Nezhat et al[18] is, to date, the largest to compare treatment by robotic-assisted laparoscopy (RALS) (40 patients) versus conventional laparoscopy (CLS) (38 patients) in patients with various stages of endometriosis. In these groups, only nine robotic surgery patients and eight conventional laparoscopy patients had severe endometriosis. It was found that robot-assisted laparoscopic and conventional laparoscopic treatment of endometriosis showed no statistically significant differences in outcomes, except for a longer operating time for the robotic surgical technique. In another retrospective cohort study, Bedaiwy et al[19] reviewed 43 cases of severe endometriosis treated with robot-assisted laparoscopy and found it to be a reasonably safe and feasible method for definitive surgical management of this condition. Siesto et al[20] published a retrospective cohort study of 43 patients with deep infiltrating endometriosis (DIE) treated by RALS, including 19 bowel resections, 23 removals of nodules from the rectovaginal septum, and 5 bladder resections; they found the robotic approach to be a safe and attractive alternative to accomplish comprehensive surgical treatment of DIE (**Fig. 7.3**).

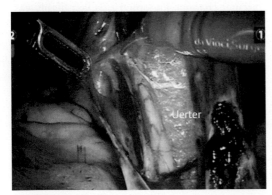

Fig. 7.1   Ureterolysis.

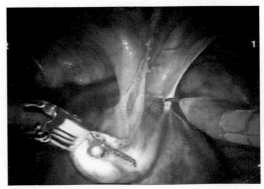

Fig. 7.2   Adhesiolysis.

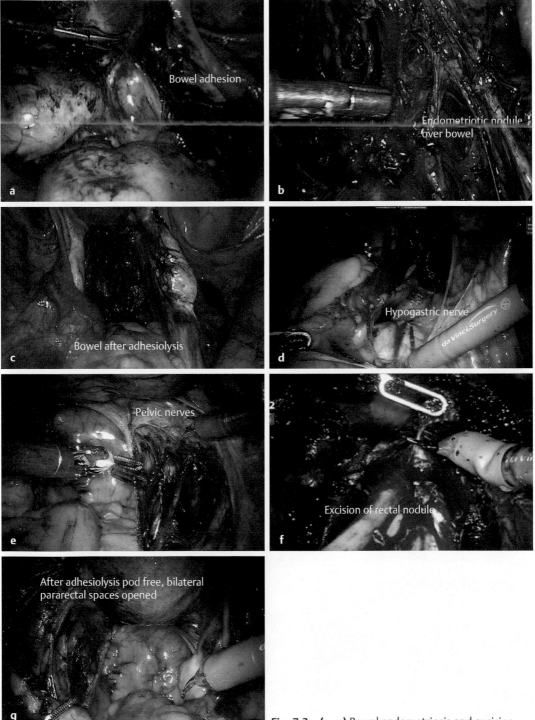

Fig. 7.3 (a–g) Bowel endometriosis and excision.

Several case reports showing the feasibility of robotic-assisted laparoscopy in cases of severe endometriosis involving the bladder, rectum, and bowel have been published. Chammas et al[21] published a case report about a 23-year-old woman with a 4cm bladder mass and rectal nodules confirmed to be endometriosis; she successfully underwent robotic-assisted laparoscopic partial cystectomy with excision of rectal nodules for endometriosis (**Fig. 7.4**). Another case report of bladder endometriosis successfully removed by RALS in a 32-year-old woman was published by Liu et al.[22] In Brazil, Averbach et al[23] published a case report in which a 35-year-old woman with DIE with rectal involvement underwent colorectal resection by use of a robot; they found it to be a safe and feasible approach. A case series published by Nezhat et al[24] showed the advantage of the RALS approach in treating five patients with multiorgan endometriosis, including ovaries, bowel, bladder, and ureteral endometriosis, concluding that robotic-assisted laparoscopy may provide the adequate platform for inexperienced laparoscopic surgeons in converting those complex procedures from the laparotomy approach to the minimally invasive approach (**Fig. 7.1** and **Figs. 7.3** to **7.5**).

In order to compare both methods of endometriosis surgery, an extensive randomized control trial (RCT) is needed with an increase in sample size.

Review of robotic endometriosis surgery at our center showed increased complexity with the majority of patients with grade 4 endometriosis undergoing surgery. Outcomes of operative time and length of stay are comparable to laparoscopy done by the same surgeon. The intraoperative complication was only one rectal serosal tear which was recognized intraoperatively and sutured. We had no conversion to laparoscopy or laparotomy. ICG dye was used to identify ureters in few cases. There was a difference in postoperative pain; paracetamol was the only analgesic used with early mobilization. Long-term follow-up showed resolution of pain with endometriosis and conception. There were no long-term complications.

Tips and tricks of using da Vinci robotic system in endometriosis surgery:

- Docking in the Si system should always be side docking as that allows the use of sound manipulation of the uterus vaginally; this enables elevation of the uterus over the pouch of Douglas and dissection of the planes.
- Port placement in the Si system is in W fashion, ensuring an 8cm gap between the ports. Xi allows ports in a single line and gives adequate access with no crowding. The assistant port is 5 mm, single port usually in upper right quadrant (**Fig. 7.6**).
- We found the use of Maryland bipolar forceps, monopolar scissors, prograsp most useful. The needle holder is seldom required in endometriosis surgery unless it is with a hysterectomy.
- Energy sources needed are bipolar and monopolar. Monopolar scissors tip is used as monopolar needle/spatula to use current for dissection. Ultrasound energy devices do not have wristed movements; hence, the usability is limited.

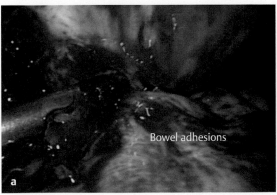 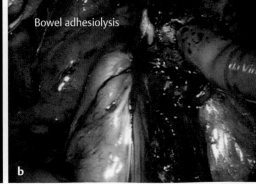

Fig. 7.4   (a, b) Adhesiolysis.

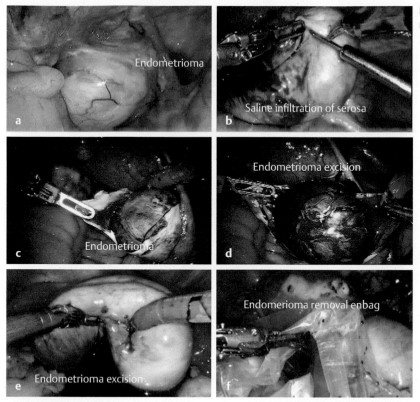

Fig. 7.5 (a–f) Endometrioma excision.

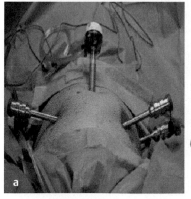

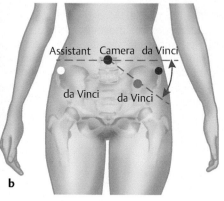

Fig. 7.6 (a, b) Port placement.

- The third arm should use the prograsp for assistance. In the case of adherent bowel, it is not advisable to use the prograsp, as manipulation can lead to serosal tears.
- ICG dye can be used to flush the ureters with a ureteric catheter and cystoscopy prior to surgical incision. In Xi robot, this helps in highlighting the ureter and its path on use of a green filter. Endometriosis surgery safety depends on lateralization of the ureter, and in most cases, it is deeply buried in adhesions. The use of ICG, though adds 10 minutes to procedure time saves significant time intraoperatively and anxiety.

- ICG has been reported to be used in DIE surgery through an IV injection. The dye takes 15 minutes to be visible in the pelvis. Vascular lesions with fibrotic tissue can be delineated and excised completely.
- Telescope used is always 0 degrees.

The efficacy of the use of robotic technology in severe endometriosis surgery is yet to be shown to be statistically significant. The lack of RCT studies and the small database used to compare the laparoscopic versus robotic approach are limitations to prove the same. A meta-analysis conducted by Restiano et al[25] showed a lack of extensive data. They analyzed five comparative studies between laparoscopy and robotic surgery, and 1527 patients were studied. They found both approaches comparable for blood loss, but complications with robotic surgery had longer operative time. The multidisciplinary surgeons needed and lack of similar cases can be the reason for this.

The cost of robotic surgery is more than laparoscopy; however, the use of multiple surgeons and complexity can justify the expense.

In conclusion, minimally invasive surgery should be considered the standard for the management of patients with endometriosis. Data from the literature showed that robotic surgery is not inferior to laparoscopy techniques, and it is safe and productive. Thanks to the three-dimensional vision with the freeness of movement of robotic instruments, robotic-assisted surgeries (RAS) allows obtaining higher surgical precision. We could consider this approach a valid alternative to standard laparoscopy, especially in deep infiltrative endometriosis with bowel and ureteral involvement; its use in patients with mild or moderate disease involving the ovaries and with superficial peritoneal involvement is limited.

References

1. Giudice LC, Kao LC. Endometriosis. Lancet 2004;364(9447):1789–1799
2. Burney RO, Giudice LC. The pathogenesis of endometriosis. In: Nezhat C, Nezhat F, Nezhat C, eds. Nezhat's video-assisted and robotic-assisted laparoscopy and hysteroscopy. 4th ed. Cambridge, England: Cambridge University Press; 2013:252–259.
3. Balasch J, Creus M, Fábregues F, et al. Visible and non-visible endometriosis at laparoscopy in fertile and infertile women and in patients with chronic pelvic pain: a prospective study. Hum Reprod 1996;11(2):387–391
4. Lucidi RS, Witz CA. Endometriosis. In: Alvero R, Schlaff WD, eds. Endocrinology and infertility: the requisites in obstetrics and gynecology. 1st ed. Philadelphia, PA: Mosby Elsevier; 2007:213–228
5. Kappou D, Matalliotakis M, Matalliotakis I. Medical treatments for endometriosis. Minerva Ginecol 2010;62(5):415–432
6. Scarselli G, Rizzello F, Cammilli F, Ginocchini L, Coccia ME. Diagnosis and treatment of endometriosis. A review. Minerva Ginecol 2005;57(1):55–78
7. Nezhat C, Bueschler E, Paka C, et al. Video-assisted laparoscopic treatment of endometriosis. In: Nezhat C, Nezhat F, Nezhat C, eds. Nezhat's video-assisted and robotic-assisted laparoscopy and hysteroscopy. 4th ed. Cambridge, England: Cambridge University Press; 2013:265–296
8. Paraiso MF, Walters MD, Rackley RR, Melek S, Hugney C. Laparoscopic and abdominal sacral colpopexies: a comparative cohort study. Am J Obstet Gynecol 2005;192(5):1752–1758
9. Mais V, Ajossa S, Guerriero S, Mascia M, Solla E, Melis GB. Laparoscopic versus abdominal myomectomy: a prospective, randomized trial to evaluate benefits in early outcome. Am J Obstet Gynecol 1996;174(2):654–658
10. Nezhat C, Crowgey SR, Garrison CP. Surgical treatment of endometriosis via laser laparoscopy. Fertil Steril 1986;45(6):778–783
11. Stylopoulos N, Rattner D. Robotics and ergonomics. Surg Clin North Am 2003;83(6):1321–1337
12. Desimone CP, Ueland FR. Gynecologic laparoscopy. Surg Clin North Am 2008;88(2):319–341, vi
13. Nezhat C, Nezhat F, Nezhat C. Operative laparoscopy (minimally invasive surgery): state of the art. J Gynecol Surg 1992;8(3):111–141
14. Nezhat C, Lavie O, Lemyre M, Unal E, Nezhat CH, Nezhat F. Robot-assisted laparoscopic surgery in gynecology: scientific dream or reality? Fertil Steril 2009;91(6):2620–2622
15. Nezhat C, Saberi NS, Shahmohamady B, Nezhat F. Robotic-assisted laparoscopy in gynecological surgery. JSLS 2006;10(3):317–320
16. Nezhat FR, Datta MS, Liu C, Chuang L, Zakashansky K. Robotic radical hysterectomy versus total laparoscopic radical hysterectomy

with pelvic lymphadenectomy for treatment of early cervical cancer. JSLS 2008;12(3): 227–237

17. Degueldre M, Vandromme J, Huong PT, Cadiere GB. Robotically assisted laparoscopic microsurgical tubal reanastomosis: a feasibility study. Fertil Steril. 2000;74(5):1020-1023.

18. Nezhat C, Lewis M, Kotikela S, et al. Robotic versus standard laparoscopy for the treatment of endometriosis. Fertil Steril 2010,94(7). 2758–2760

19. Bedaiwy MA, Rahman MY, Chapman M, et al. Robotic-assisted hysterectomy for the management of severe endometriosis: a retrospective review of short-term surgical outcomes. JSLS 2013;17(1):95–99

20. Siesto G, Ieda N, Rosati R, Vitobello D. Robotic surgery for deep endometriosis: a paradigm shift. Int J Med Robot 2014;10(2):140–146

21. Chammas MF Jr, Kim FJ, Barbarino A, et al. Asymptomatic rectal and bladder endometriosis: a case for robotic-assisted surgery. Can J Urol 2008;15(3):4097–4100

22. Liu C, Perisic D, Samadi D, Nezhat F. Robotic-assisted laparoscopic partial bladder resection for the treatment of infiltrating endometriosis. J Minim Invasive Gynecol 2008;15(6):745–748

23. Averbach M, Popoutchi P, Marques OW Jr, Abdalla RZ, Podgaec S, Abrão MS. Robotic rectosigmoidectomy: pioneer case report in Brazil. Current scene in colorectal robotic surgery. Arq Gastroenterol 2010;47(1): 116–118

24. Nezhat C, Hajhosseini B, King LP. Robotic-assisted laparoscopic treatment of bowel, bladder, and ureteral endometriosis. JSLS 2011;15(3):387–392

25. Restaino S, Mereu L, Finelli A, et al. Robotic surgery vs laparoscopic surgery in patients with diagnosis of endometriosis: a systematic review and meta-analysis. J Robot Surg 2020; 14(5):687–694

Accompanying Video

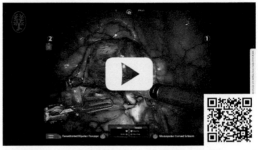

Video 7.1   Endometriosis. https://www.thieme.de/ de/q.htm?p=opn/cs/21/6/15245533-06864b0d

8 Robotic Vesicovaginal Fistula

Ankur Mittal and Indira Sarin

Introduction and Definition

A fistula can be defined as an extra-anatomic communication between two or more epithelial- and mesothelial-lined surfaces. When this abnormal communication is between urinary and genital tracts, it forms a urogenital fistula. A patient with continuous urinary leakage is distressed and has detrimental impact on her quality of life and is also socially stigmatized in most circumstances. Such is the fate of this social problem that active intervention in surgical repair is almost always needed. These reconstructions are often complex, and it becomes essential for the operating surgeon to be well versed in various techniques and approaches. One such state-of-the-art technique is the robot-assisted laparoscopic repair of genitourinary fistula. Its excellent outcomes, backed by minimal morbidity and complications, are promising management options for women suffering from this highly distressing disease.

Types and Etiology

The most common acquired fistula of the urinary tract is the vesicovaginal fistula (VVF). Other urinary fistulae are ureterovaginal (UVF), urethrovaginal, vesicocervical, ureterocervical, vesicouterine, and ureterouterine. The prevalence and etiology of fistulae vary between the developing and developed nations. In the developing world, VVF is most common (>75%) and mainly forms after an obstetric misadventure. In developed countries, VVF is most commonly caused due to bladder injury at the time of any pelvic surgery like gynecologic, urologic, or others. **Table 8.1** enumerates the etiology of VVF.

Classifications

- Depending on the clinical examination—vesicocervical, juxtacervical, midvaginal vesicovaginal, suburethral vesicovaginal, and urethrovaginal.
- Depending on the size of VVF—small <2 cm, medium 2 to 3 cm, large 4 to 5 cm, and extensive >6 cm.
- Depending on the site—supratrigonal, trigonal, and infratrigonal (bladder neck).
- Depending on complexity—(a) Simple: <2 to 3 cm, single tract, supratrigonal, no previous history of malignancy or radiation, normal vaginal length, surrounded by healthy tissues with good accessibility. (b) Complex: >3 cm, multiple tracts, trigonal or below, history of previous attempt of repair or malignancy or radiation, recurrent, one with short vaginal length, involving urethra, bladder neck, ureter, or intestines.
- Depending on the etiology—congenital and acquired. Acquired VVF can be subdivided as malignant, benign, traumatic, infective/inflammatory, and miscellaneous.
- Depending on the involvement of continent mechanism—(a) Type 1: Not involving the closing mechanism; (b) Type 2: Involving the closing mechanism: (i) not involving total urethra, (ii) involving total urethra; and (c) Type 3: Miscellaneous, (viz., ureteric fistula).
- The classification system makes it easier for a clinician to categorize the fistulae and hence decide upon the further course or route of treatment and their follow-up,

Table 8.1 Etiology of vesicovaginal fistula

Sl. No.	Causes	
1.	Iatrogenic	• Hysterectomy—abdominal/vaginal • Anterior vaginal wall prolapse surgery (colporrhaphy) • Anti-incontinence procedures • Vaginal biopsy • Bladder biopsy, endoscopic resection, laser therapy • Other pelvic surgeries (vascular, rectal)
2.	Obstetric	• Obstructed labor • Injury during instrumental delivery (forceps) • Rupture of uterus • Bladder injury during caesarean section
3.	External traumatic	• Pelvic fracture, penetrating, sexual, female genital mutilation
4.	Radiation induced	
5.	Advanced pelvic malignancy	• Bladder, rectal, cervical tumors
6.	Infection or inflammation	• Tuberculosis, STD, schistosomiasis
7.	Foreign body	• Forgotten vaginal pessary, sex toys, herbs, cups
8.	Congenital	• Associated with other genitourinary anomalies
9.	Others	• Tobacco abuse, diabetes mellitus, poverty, malnourishment, contracted pelvis

although we cannot determine the outcome of a particular treatment based on these systems.

Clinical Presentation

Patients most commonly complain of continuous urinary leak from the vagina. Amount of leak may be variable and usually corresponds to the size of fistula. Self-voiding may be present based on the site and size of fistula and the volume of urinary leakage. This leak may be positional, minimal while lying and increasing manifolds while standing. VVF must be distinguished from other causes of urinary leak per vaginam, like urinary incontinence, stress or urgency, overflow incontinence, ureterovaginal fistula.

The manifestation of leak per vaginam usually occurs after 1 to 3 weeks of a traumatic surgical event, or after removing the urethral catheter. A radiation fistula manifests late and may take even

months to years after completion of radiation. Other associated findings may involve amenorrhea, PID, lower limb contractures following nerve injury, foot drop secondary to sacral and perineal nerve compression, and neurogenic bladder dysfunction.

Evaluation and Diagnosis

A thorough history with complete examination usually aids in the diagnosis (**Fig. 8.1**).

Local pelvic examination may reveal vulvar excoriations and ammoniacal dermatitis.

Pooling of fluid in the vagina may be seen, which, when followed by a careful per speculum examination of the entire anterior vaginal wall, may reveal the fistula. An assessment of the location, size, number of fistulae, condition of surrounding tissue, tissue mobility, vaginal access to the fistular site, any associated rectovaginal fistula is made. A bimanual examination with

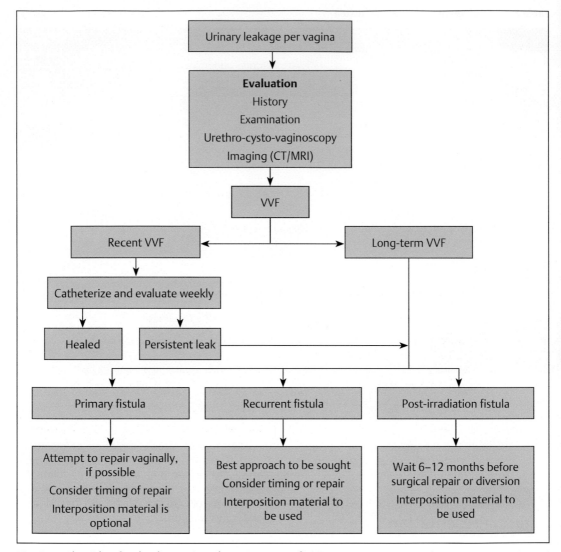

Fig. 8.1   Algorithm for the diagnosis and management of VVF.

careful palpation of the anterior wall or filling the bladder with a dyed solution per urethra and then examining the anterior vaginal wall may help locate the fistula in cases of small or occult fistulae. In certain cases, three swab test/tampon test of Moir or a double dye test may be required, where the vagina is packed with gauze pieces and their differential staining with dye filled in bladder determines the site of fistula.

Cystovaginoscopy: An endourological evaluation of the bladder and vagina with a modified endoscope or a flexible cystoscope reveals the precise location of the fistulous tract, its size, distance from the ureteric orifices, any collateral fistulae, etc.

Imaging: VVF is associated with ureteral injury or ureterovaginal fistula in 10 to 12% of cases; hence, an evaluation of the upper urinary tract is important. A contrast computed tomography (CT) or magnetic resonance imaging (MRI) is generally performed. In cases where they aren't available, IVU or VCUG with upper tract study can be performed alternatively.

Other tests: urinalysis and culture, serum creatinine levels, creatinine levels in the pooled vaginal fluid may be adjunctive tests.

Treatment

The Conservative Treatment

The options for conservative treatment are mentioned in the chart in **Fig. 8.2**.

However, such therapy is suitable only for carefully selected cases with the following indication:

- Progressively reducing urinary leak with catheterization.
- New-onset fistula <3 weeks.
- Narrow fistula tract with size <1 cm.

Surgical Repair (Fig. 8.3)

The initial attempt is the best time to achieve a successful repair, owing to the hindrance caused by anatomic distortions and fibrosis in subsequent attempts.

The timing of repair is still controversial; however, optimal timing targeted toward minimizing patient's sufferings should be sought. The traditional teaching recommendations of a 3 to 6 months delay have waned. The delay is warranted only in cases of radiation-induced fistulas, because of severe endarteritis obliterans and jeopardized tissue vascularity. In cases of obstructed labor, a waiting period of 3 to 6 months is optimum to allow for the edema and inflammation to subside. Uncomplicated postsurgical urinary fistulae may be repaired as soon as diagnosed.

Route of repair is often influenced by the size, location, need for concomitant procedures, and expertise of the operating surgeon. **Table 8.2** enumerates the indications/advantages and contraindications of each route.

Commandments of Surgical Repair of a Urinary Fistula

- Adequately exposing the fistulous tract by debriding the necrosed and ischemic tissue.
- Any synthetic/foreign bodies need to be removed from the fistular region, if applicable.
- Cautiously separating the involved organ cavities by meticulous dissection.
- Achieving watertight closure.
- Nontraumatic tissue handling to facilitate the availability of healthy and vascular tissue flaps.

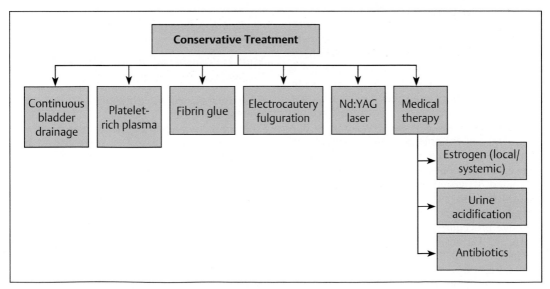

Fig. 8.2 Conservative treatment.

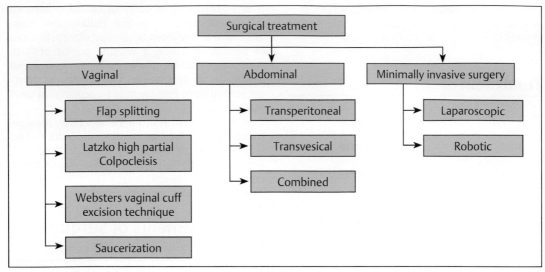

Fig. 8.3 Surgical repair.

- Multiple-layer closure with nonoverlapping suture lines.
- Anastomosis should be tension-free.
- To achieve satisfactory urinary tract drainage and/or stenting after repair.
- To treat and prevent infections by judicious use of appropriate antimicrobials.
- To achieve and maintain hemostasis.

Robotic Repair of VVF

Employing the best of technology to foster the benefits in the medical field is a boon to humanity and one such state-of-the-art advantage is the sophisticated robotic systems. The robotic approach to surgery is a sheer amalgamation of minimally invasive approach with the dexterity and precision of an open surgery. Not only this, the overall patient outcomes are better in terms of success rates, decreased morbidity, and faster recovery. The robot is equipped with a highly magnified 3D vision and a 360-degree endowrist which gives ease of operation to the console surgeon, even in such types of challenging reconstructive procedures in deep pelvis that require severe angulations.

Preoperative patient counseling: However, before embarking on the surgical repair, thorough patient counseling is a must, carefully explaining the successful outcomes as well as failures,

and also the need of prolonged catheterization. A short-term, self-limited postoperative episode of urinary urgency and frequency may occur after removal of the catheter. Finally, the need of interpositional flaps or grafts may occur, and it must be made clear to the patient that various intraoperative factors may alter the surgical plan during operation (**Table 8.3**).

Melamund described the first successful robotic repair in 2005.

Operative Steps

Step 1: Positioning of the Patient and Preliminary Cystoscopy

Patient is placed in lithotomy position under general anesthesia.

Examination using a cystoscope is performed and ureters are catheterized if needed. A ureteral catheter is also placed across the fistula and taken out through the vagina. A urethral catheter is placed. Now after securing the patient with belts and shoulder bolsters, a low lithotomy position is given.

Step 2: Port Placement and Docking

After creating pneumoperitoneum, a 12-mm primary/camera port is made supraumbilical. Three 8-mm robotic ports are placed 8 cm apart: two on

Table 8.2 Vaginal and abdominal routes of repair

Sl. no.	Route of surgery	Indications	Advantages	Contraindications
1.	Vaginal	1. Abdominal wall scarring by previous surgery	1. No need of bladder or abdominal incisions 2. Repair can be undertaken immediately	1. Narrow, inaccessible, and scarred vagina
		2. Primary route of repair for uncomplicated fistula with easy vaginal access	3. Multiple interposition flap options, labial fat pad (martius), peritoneal, gracilis myocutaneous flap, gluteal skin flap	2. Coexistent rectovaginal fistula
			4. Shorter operative time	3. Radiation fistulae
			5. Less blood loss	
			6. Shorter hospital stay	
			7. Lesser morbidity and quicker recovery	
			8. Reimplantation may not be necessary even if fistula tract is near the ureteric orifice	
			9. Lower cost	
2.	Abdominal	1. Preferred when vaginal route cannot be used, has failed, or is inaccessible, (e.g., high fistula with narrow vagina)	No risk of vaginal shortening; hence, sexual functions are not affected	
		2. Complicated fistulae requiring ancillary procedures like ureteric reimplantation and augmentation cystoplasty		
		3. Presence of vesical stones		
		4. Postradiation fistula		
		5. When patient cannot be put in a lithotomy position		

Table 8.3   Equipment for robotic VVF repair

Robotic instruments
• Three 8-mm trocars • A 0-degree and 30-degree three-dimensional (3D) laparoscope • Hot Shears (monopolar curved scissors) • Maryland Bipolar Forceps • One large needle driver and one SutureCut needle driver • ProGrasp Forceps
Laparoscopic equipment
• One trocar (12 mm) bedside assistant • One 5-mm trocar (bedside assistant) (optional) • A 5-mm suction cannula • A 5-mm laparoscopic grasper • A 5-mm endoscopic needle driver
Suture materials
• 3–0 Poliglecaprone monofilament synthetic absorbable suture • 3–0 Barbed suture (polyglyconate)

left paramedian and left far lateral sides and one on the right paramedian side. Vagina is packed with a sponge. Robot is thereafter docked, putting the patient in steep Trendelenburg position.

Step 3: Peritoneoscopy and Adhesiolysis

An extensive adhesiolysis of the omentum and bowel is performed using sharp and blunt dissection.

Step 4: Posterior Minicystostomy

Fistula is localized and the bladder is vertically incised on its posterior wall, close to the VVF (**Fig. 8.4**).

Step 5: Excision of Fistula and Necrotic Tissue

Resected margins of the fistula are carefully excised and the tissue is sent for histopathology (**Fig. 8.5**).

Step 6: Separation of the Bladder from the Vagina

Flaps of the bladder and vagina are raised and after meticulous dissection the two organ cavities are mobilized off each other (**Fig. 8.6**).

Step 7: Reconstruction of Vagina

Vagina is closed in a tension-free manner using a 3–0 barbed or Vicryl as a running watertight suture (**Fig. 8.7**).

Step 8: Placement of Interposition Tissue

A well-vascularized healthy pedicle of omentum, peritoneum, or epiploicae of the sigmoid colon may be used to interpose between the vagina and the bladder (**Fig. 8.8**).

Step 9: Bladder Closure

Bladder closure is done in preferably two layers using a 3–0 barbed suture. A watertight tension-free closure is ensured (**Fig. 8.9**).

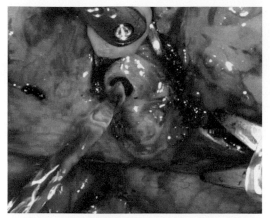

Fig. 8.4 Cystostomy.

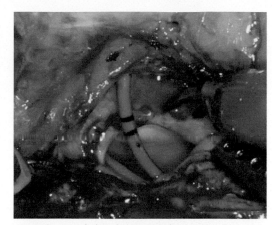

Fig. 8.5 Fistula localization and excision.

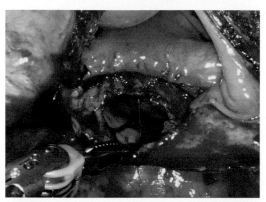

Fig. 8.6 Separation of bladder and vagina.

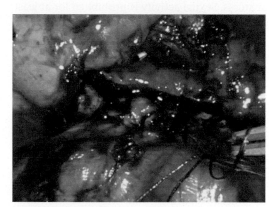

Fig. 8.7 Closure of vagina.

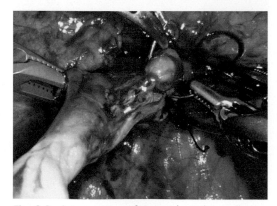

Fig. 8.8 Interposition of sigmoid epiploicae flap.

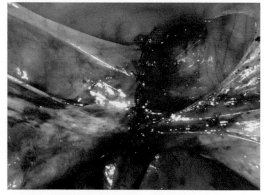

Fig. 8.9 Bladder closure.

Step 10: Drain Placement, Deflation of Peritoneum, Trocar Removal, and Skin Closure

Postoperative Care

Proper antibiotic coverage is advised postoperatively. Early ambulation is also advised. Liquid diet can be started the same evening followed by normal diet the next day. The abdominal drain is typically removed after 24 hours of surgery. Care of urethral catheter is advised on discharge. The catheter is to be kept for 2 to 3 weeks and removed under antibiotic cover. Anticholinergics may be required for bladder spasms. Patients are advised to avoid heavy exercises and straining at stools. Sexual activity is prohibited for at least 8 weeks.

Outcomes of Robotic VVF

Robotic VVF repair is an efficacious and safe technique in trained hands, with the following advantages: Three-dimensional vision and superior depth perception, termer filtration, motion scaling, 10× magnification, and endowrist with 7-degree mobility leading to enhanced dexterity and absence of fatigue, which contribute to precise reconstruction. Major complication rate of 2.3% has been reported, which includes compartment syndrome in lower extremities, enterocutaneous fistula, and inferior epigastric artery injury. When compared to laparoscopic or open repair, it has shown to have improved success rates and reduced morbidity. The high cost of robotic VVF repair is a major limitation to its routine use; however, it is a brilliant option for otherwise difficult to manage, recurrent fistulas.

Suggested Reading

Badlani GH, De Ridder JMKD, Reddy MJ, Rovner ES. Campbell-Walsh-Wein urology. 11 ed. Philadelphia, PA: Elsevier; 2016. Chapter 89, 2103

De Ridder JMKD, Greenwell T. Campbell-Walsh-Wein urology. 11 ed. Philadelphia, PA: Elsevier; 2016: Chapter 129, 2924

Gupta NP, Mishra S, Hemal AK, Mishra A, Seth A, Dogra PN. Comparative analysis of outcome between open and robotic surgical repair of recurrent supra-trigonal vesico-vaginal fistula. J Endourol 2010;24(11):1779–1782

Rajaian S, Pragatheeswarane M, Panda A. Vesicovaginal fistula: review and recent trends. Indian J Urol 2019;35(4):250–258

Accompanying Video

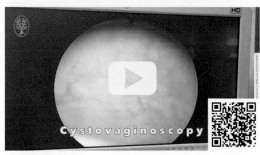

Video 8.1   Robot-assisted VVF repair. https://www.thieme.de/de/q.htm?p=opn/cs/21/6/15245408-87285243

9 Concept of Sentinel Lymph Node Biopsy in Gynecological Cancers

Anupama Rajanbabu and Madhavi Dokku

Introduction

Regional lymphadenectomy is an integral part of comprehensive staging in gynecological malignancies,[1,2] which despite having debatable therapeutic benefit[3–5] has important role in prognostication, staging, and in tailoring the adjuvant treatment beyond any doubt.[2,6,7]

However, conventional lymphadenectomy is brimmed with perioperative complications such as the risk of vascular, nerve, and ureteric injury along with increase in operative time, infections, and vascular thrombosis. In addition, there is an increase in overall cost and long-term complications such as neuralgia, lower extremity lymphedema, and lymphocele, all affecting quality of life (QoL) of cancer survivors.[8–10] In this context, exploration on promising less-invasive novel techniques for nodal assessment unlatched the concept of sentinel lymph node biopsy (SLNB).[11,12]

History

Two decades later, from 1960, following the first description of sentinel lymph node (SLN) in parotid carcinoma by Gould et al,[13] Ramon Cabanas pioneered a groundbreaking work on sentinel node biopsy in penile cancer in 1977.[14] However, the procedure gained popularity when Morton innovated the use of blue dye for sentinel node mapping in cutaneous melanoma in 1992.[15] Giuliano et al in 1994 used vital dye with ultrastaging of sentinel nodes in breast cancer.[16] Both works are considered as pillars to the current practice of SLNB as the standard of care in the management of melanoma and breast cancer.[17,18]

This concept of SLNB in gynecological malignancies was similarly explored first in vulvar cancer by Levenback et al in 1994,[19] subsequently was applied in endometrial cancer by Burke et al in 1996,[20] and was soon extended to cervical cancer by Echt et al in 1999.[21] Since then, after multiple research works, it is now widely approved in managing vulvar cancer[22] and has recently gained heightened acceptance in the management of endometrial and early cervical cancers.[23–25]

Concepts of Sentinel Node Biopsy

A sentinel node is defined as the first node in a lymphatic basin for an anatomical region to which metastatic disease will spread first from the primary tumor.[13] This implies that if the sentinel node is negative for metastasis, the remaining nodes in the nodal basin will also be negative; hence, complete lymph node dissection can be obviated (**Fig. 9.1**).[26] Apart from decreasing the surgical morbidity,[11] added benefits noted with SLNB are localization of aberrant lymphatic pathways which are often missed during routine lymphadenectomy[27,28] and focused pathological analysis with ultrastaging and immunohistochemical staining (IHC) for cytokeratin, leading to increase in the detection rate of metastatic disease through SLNB.[29,30]

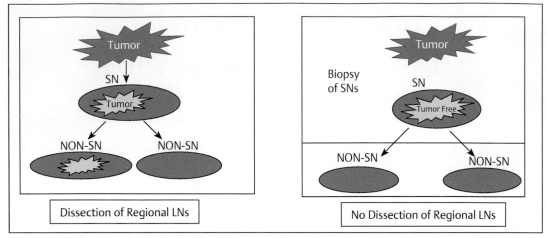

Fig. 9.1   Concept of sentinel lymph node biopsy.

Description of Technique and Tracers

A tracer is used for mapping the sentinel nodes and is injected peritumorally, then sentinel nodes are mapped and removed at the time of surgery. These nodes are sent for pathological analysis. Intraoperative frozen analysis to avoid reoperation is limited by high false-negative rate and has added risk of losing tissue for final pathological analysis; therefore, it is not considered indispensable.[31–33]

The mapping substances used in gynecological cancers include blue dyes (methylene blue, isosulfan blue) and radioisotopes (technetium 99/Tc-99) alone or in combinations[34,35] (**Fig. 9.2**).

Blue dyes are less expensive, but cause skin and urine discoloration, decrease pulse oximetry readings, paradoxical methhemoglobinemia, and rarely anaphylaxis. They are simple to use and are injected just before mapping as the dye will reach the nodes in just 5 to 10 minutes, staining lymphatics and nodes blue, which are identified directly by naked eyes. The dye soon vanishes or travel further into nonsentinel second node; hence, delay in exploration for SLN leads to failed or false nodal mapping.[36,37]

Radioisotopes have a better safety profile with very low risk of radiation exposure but are expensive and complex to use.[38] The timing of injection and nodal mapping varies with the type of protocol used. They are usually injected 2 to 24 hours before surgery. Tracers are supposed to reach the nodes in 1 to 120 minutes[39] and disintegrate within 24 hours. Nodal mapping can be done preoperatively with lymphoscintigraphy (LSG)/Single-Photon Emission Computed Tomography (SPECT) or intraoperatively from audiometric signals emitted from gamma probe in proportion to the radioactivity of the tracer.[34,40]

In recent times, indocyanine green (ICG) has been the most frequently used tracer due to its superior overall and bilateral sentinel node detection rates compared to traditional tracers, particularly in obese patients.[41] It is sterile, nontoxic, water-soluble tricarbocyanine, safe, and also Food and Drug Administration (FDA) approved; however, caution is a need in patients with iodine allergies as it contains 5% iodide. It displays fluorescence when exposed to near-infrared (NIR) light delivered by a dedicated optical system (NIR imager during laparoscopy or firefly technology during robotics); hence, sentinel nodes are easily detected by real-time fluorescent images during surgery (**Fig. 9.2**). This technology has additional assets of high penetration and low autofluorescence. ICG is injected just before surgery as it quickly travels through lymphatics without losing intensity. Hence, detection for SLN should not be delayed beyond 10 minutes and limit the detection to 25 to 30 minutes for

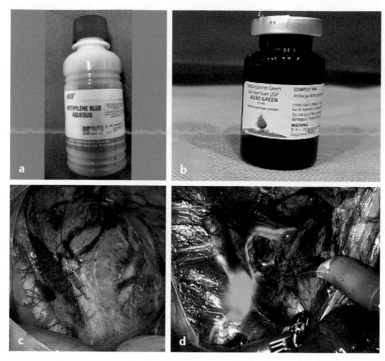

Fig. 9.2 Tracers and lymphatic mapping. **(a)** Methylene blue dye. **(b)** Left external iliac sentinel node mapped with blue dye. **(c)** Indocyanine green dye. **(d)** Left external iliac sentinel node mapped with ICG.

the risk of sampling too many nodes. At present, there is no consensus on the ideal concentration and volume of the ICG dye to be injected for the best results. All the traces have acceptable detection rates, and ICG fares well among them but it is costly and needs specific optical systems for use.[33,37,42–44]

Surgical approaches used for sentinel node mapping show a paradigm shift from open to minimally invasive laparoscopy and robotics when available.[45,46]

Ultrastaging of Sentinel Nodes

Giuliano and colleagues in 1995 first reported ultrastaging of sentinel nodes in breast cancer,[16] which is one of the most important advances in the SLNB technique.[47] It involves a histological examination of SLN by serial sectioning of node perpendicular to its long axis and wholly submitting it for hematoxylin and eosin (H&E) staining, and if no metastasis (mainly macrometastasis,

tumor >2 mm in diameter)[48] is identified, immunohistochemistry (IHC) staining with anti-pan cytokeratin antibody (AE1/AE3) is used to increase the sensitivity of the procedure. The sectioning and pathological assessment of SLN ultrastaging is shown in **Fig. 9.3**.

The advantage of ultrastaging comes from the increased detection rate of metastasis compared to routine H&E analysis.[49] This is by identification of micrometastases (μM) (0.2–2.0 mm in diameter) and isolated tumor cell (ITC) metastases (<0.2 mm in diameter, up to 200 cells)[48] which are missed on routine H&E slides. The advantage of detecting this low-volume disease (μM and ITC) is not always clear, although μM are reported to be associated with increased risk of recurrences and warrant adjuvant therapy.[50,51]

Advances in ultrastaging include the application of more sensitive techniques like quantitative reverse transcriptase-polymerase chain reaction (qRT-PCR)/OSNA (one-step nucleic assay amplification) assay for detecting CK19 mRNA to improve the intraoperative frozen diagnostic accuracy.[52]

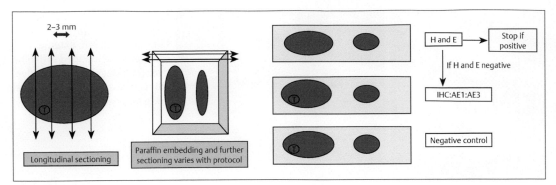

Fig. 9.3   Sentinel lymph node ultra staging concept.

Role of Sentinel Node Biopsy in Endometrial Cancer

Dispute on therapeutic benefit of complete pelvic and aortic lymphadenectomy in early endometrial cancer recommended following the reports of two randomized control studies showing no survival benefit, despite few reports of improved survival with nodal dissection in high-risk histologies.[3,4,53] But its role in staging and prognostication and deciding on the adjuvant therapy[54,55] is definitive.[9,11] Currently, a wide variation of surgical practices on nodal dissection, ranging from no nodal evaluation and associated increased use of external beam radiation[54] to comprehensive aortopelvic lymphadenectomy, are seen.[56,57]

In this scenario, SLNB appears as middle-ground option and is increasingly being adopted, with multiple reports showing promising results on feasibility with less morbidity.[58] This also seems reasonable in high-risk histologies to avoid morbidity due to frequent use of adjuvants in their management.[56] NCCN guidelines endorse sentinel node biopsy as an alternative to comprehensive lymphadenectomy in uterine-confined endometrial carcinoma but with caution because of low-level evidence.[59]

Among all the tracers available, ICG is rapidly becoming the option of choice when available, given the highest overall and bilateral detection rates.[60,61] Among the uterine fundal, hysteroscopic-guided endometrial and cervical stromal injection sites, cervical injection is the most accepted modality due its ease and reproducibility and higher detection rates of 89% and sensitivity of 84% and negative predictive value (NPV)

of 97%.[35,58,61–63] Disadvantage is its likelihood of missing para-aortic nodes.[33,62,64–66] This, however, appears to be insignificant because the risk of isolated aortic lymph node metastasis in the absence of pelvic nodal metastasis even in high-risk histology is not greater than 5%.[67–69] Adopting sentinel node mapping makes surgery less challenging in obese cohorts, who represent a substantial risk group for endometrial cancer.[70,71]

Concepts on the utility of SLNB became more evident from multi-institutional prospective studies SENTI ENDO[35] and FIRES.[72] Both the studies performed systematic pelvic with or without para-aortic lymphadenectomy after SLNB. Their outcomes disclosed detection rates of 89% and 86%, NPV of 97% and 99.6%, and sensitivity of 84% and 97.2% for detection of nodal metastasis, respectively. A recent report of pooled averages mentioned in meta-analysis on SLNB in endometrial cancer by Bodurtha Smith et al[73] showed overall detection rates of 81% and bilateral detection rate of 50%, and sensitivity of 96% for detection of SLN metastasis.

Factors needed for optimizing detection rates noted in previous studies include surgeon's experience, application of structured systemic algorithm as proposed by Barlin et al,[74] use of ultrastaging,[47] intracervical tracer injection,[62] use of ICG dye,[61] and laparoscopic or robotic approach.[65,75]

From a growing body of evidence showing low false-negative SLNB rates, it can be concluded that it is appropriate for low-risk histology. Future trials should concentrate on the benefit of increased detection of low-volume disease through ultrastaging and clarify the role of SLNB in high-risk groups.

Role of Sentinel Node Biopsy in Cervical Cancer

Standard care for operable early stage cervical cancer includes systematic bilateral pelvic lymphadenectomy along with radical hysterectomy or trachelectomy[76–78] for its obvious benefits in prognostication,[6,79–82] Added node positivity indicates the need for adjuvant treatment[83] and upstages the disease.[84]

However, the possibility of node positivity in early cervical cancer is 15 to 31%,[29,78,85–88] suggesting the majority undergo lymphadenectomy[10] with no benefit. Also, because of complex lymphatic drainage[89] of the cervix, definitive prediction of the site of metastatic aberrant pathways of spread[27,28] can be difficult, which can be better detected with SLNB.

Research describes two or four quadrants cervical stromal injection[90–93] of blue dyes[21,91] and radioisotopes,[94–96] both alone or in combination,[97–99] reporting detection rates of 84%, 88%, 97%, respectively.[100] Efforts to improve localization of sentinel node with preoperative LSG along with radioactive tracers were not very affirmative; however, in comparison, SPECT offered significant improvement in detection rates.[101–103]

Traditional techniques of SLNB report overall sentinel node detection rates of 88 to 98% and bilateral detection rates of 59 to 76%, sensitivity for detection of metastases of 77.4 to 92%, and a negative predictive value of 94.3 to 98%.[23,96,97,104] The most extensive retrospective study published by Cibula et al reported sensitivity of 91% in the whole cohort, with 97% in bilateral sentinel node biopsy cohort and a false-negative rate of 2.8% with ultrastaging.[49]

Approaches can be either by laparoscopy[45] or laparotomy.[92,105] However, the newer technique ICG-NIF using robotic platform reports the highest performance.[46]

It is imperative to include ultrastaging with SLNB to decrease false-negative rate[49] through increased detection of μM and ITC.[51] Retrospective studies also consider μM diagnosed during ultrastaging as an independent prognostic factor of survival,[106–108] encouraging the use of adjuvant radiation in their management.

Use of intraoperative frozen for one-step approach to triage node-positive patients to primary chemoradiation or abort radical trachelectomy or conization appears incentivizing but is limited by a high false-negative rate of 30 to 50%,[31,32,109] with an additional risk of losing nodal tissue for further pathological processing.

SENTICOL study[97] mentions an overall detection rate of 95% and bilateral detection rate of 76%, an overall sensitivity of 92%, NPV of 98.2%, with false-negative rate of 0%, and 100% sensitivity in bilateral node detection cases. Other studies also confirm the feasibility and diagnostic usefulness of SLNB in early cervical cancer.[110–112] However, evidence on oncological safety is limited, and ongoing SENTICOL III and SENTIX trials, both evaluating safety as their primary endpoint, might provide more insights.

SLN mapping can be optimized by tracer combination, restricting use of SLNB to tumors <2 cm,[104] bilateral SLN detection and strict use of sentinel node algorithm proposed by Cormier et al,[112] laparoscopic approach, increased surgeons experience, and ultrastaging of sentinel nodes, excluding cases with prior neoadjuvant chemotherapy (NACT) as it may decrease the detection rates. Prior cervical conization, however, is not associated with inferior results.[113] Challenges in tracing SLN in parametrium, which may contain 8% metastatic node, can be overcome by an en-bloc parametrectomy.[114]

To conclude, despite not being included as the standard of care, a paradigm shift is noted toward SLN biopsy in clinical practice from a growing body of evidence supporting it. NCCN and 2017 ESGO/ESTRO/ESP guidelines[115,116] endorse SLNB as an alternative to complete pelvic lymphadenectomy in early cervical cancer.

Surgical Algorithm for SLNB in Cervical and Endometrial Cancer

Lymphatic drainage from uterine corpus and cervix is complex and bilateral.[89] Ipsilateral nodal status of hemipelvis is not representative of opposite side hemipelvis; therefore, unilateral sentinel node detection is insufficient and adds to a false-negative rate.

Cormier et al[112] from their retrospective analysis developed a simple systematic algorithm for SLNB in early cervical cancer which includes removal of all mapped nodes, if mapping fails to do side-specific complete nodal dissection including interiliac or subaortic nodes along with removal of any suspicious nodes if present, regardless of mapping and en-bloc parametrectomy along with primary tumor.

Similarly, Barlin et al[74] proposed an algorithm for SLN biopsy in endometrial cancer which includes peritoneal and serosal evaluation and washings, removal of all mapped nodes, if mapping fails to do side-specific completed pelvic lymphadenectomy and para-aortic lymphadenectomy with attending discretion, along with removal of suspicious nodes if present regardless of mapping. This is also recommended by NCCN guidelines.[59]

The rationale for removing abnormal nodes is that they may represent the de facto sentinel nodes not mapped or may increase the risk of harboring metastasis.[74,112]

Role of Sentinel Node Biopsy in Vulvar Cancer

Nodal status in vulvar cancer is the most important prognostic factor,[117,118] and inguinofemoral lymph node dissection (IFLND) is contemplated in the surgical management of early stage vulvar squamous cell carcinoma (SCC) with >1 mm depth of invasion.[119,120] It is associated with complications like wound infection, wound break down, lymphocele, and risk of lower limb lymphedema in almost 30% leading to reduced QoL.[121,122]

Hence, based on the outcomes of the Groningen International Study on Sentinel nodes in Vulvar cancer (GROINSS-V)[123] and Gynecological Oncology Group (GOG)-173 study,[124] SLNB in invasive SCC vulva is accepted as standard of care in selected cases of apparent early stage vulvar cancer which is also accredited by NCCN guidelines.[125]

Candidates for SLNB are patients with unifocal tumors <4 cm and clinically/radiologically absent suspicious groin nodes. Best setting and technique for SLNB includes competent surgeon working in high-volume cancer center, use of dual tracer for sentinel node mapping (blue dye and Tc-99 sulfur colloid), four-quadrant peritumoral intradermal injections, and inclusion of ultrastaging protocol for pathological analysis of SLN.[125,126]

Based on the basics of the lymphatic pathways of the vulva, midline lesions need bilateral mapping, and if lesion is >2 cm from midline, ipsilateral sentinel node biopsy is sufficient. If mapping fails, complete ipsilateral lymphadenectomy should be performed.[125] If the sentinel node is positive, complete inguinofemoral lymphadenectomy is most commonly recommended.[127]

Recent advances on improvising the technique of SLNB in vulvar cancer using SPECT and novel IGC-NIF imaging technique with the robotic platform are showing promising results and require further evaluation.[128,129]

Role of Sentinel Node Biopsy in Vaginal Cancer

Data on lymph node dissection and SLNB in vaginal cancer are insufficient; hence, their role in management is unclear, and FIGO staging is still clinical. First report on SLNB in vaginal cancer by Frumovitz et al[130] reported a presurgical sentinel detection rate of 79%. The most common mapping technique used is combination tracers, with peritumoral injection of Tc-99 followed by preoperative mapping using LSG and intraoperative sentinel node detection with blue dye and gamma probe.[131] In conclusion, though not the standard of care, studies are ongoing to improve its efficacy, and more studies are looking into outcomes of SPECT for better image accusation.[132,133]

Role of Sentinel Node Biopsy in Ovarian Cancer

SLN detection in ovarian cancer has limited evidence, with more experience seen with combination mapping using Tc-99 and blue dye and recently ICG with fluorescent tracer.[134] The injection site is debatable and includes the hilum of ovaries, both ovarian ligaments and ovarian capsules.[135,136] The broadcast detection rate is 84%[137]; however, its benefit in the clinical application should be further looked into by extensive multicentric studies to consider SLNB in ovarian cancer management.

Role of Robotic Surgery in SLNB of Gynec Cancers

Robotic surgery in gynecological oncology has seen a rapid surge since its clearance by FDA in 2005. This is due to its technical advantage over conventional laparoscopy along with the benefits of laparoscopy. With apparently short learning curve along with oncological safety and added advantage of overcoming the practical challenges of obesity and elderly with comorbidities, it is frequently used for pelvic and aortic lymphadenectomy and SLNB procedures.[70,71,138]

Introduction of firefly technology in da Vinci Xi Surgical System (Intuitive Surgical, Sunnyvale, CA) eased the use of ICG-NIF imaging technique for SLNB in endometrial cancers and cervical cancers, recently found to be less invasive and feasible in vulvar cancer and appears encouraging to research into for ovarian cancers also.[46,129]

Since Rossi et al's[72] pilot work, a number of reports have confirmed superior outcomes of this technique. Preliminary studies on this technique in the Indian setting by Rajanbabu et al reported the feasibility and high overall detection rates of 90% and bilateral detection rates of 72% even in the learning curve period.[139] The FIRES trial[75] in endometrial cancer, as mentioned before, using this technique, detected at least one sentinel node in 86% of cases, and sensitivity to detect node positive disease was 97.2% and reported a very high NPV of 99.6%. Thus, it can be stated robotics increases the overall detection rate. A recent meta-analysis of 17 articles including 1059 patients by Wu et al[140] on this technique reports detection rates ranging from 76 to 100% with a pooled average of 95%, and sensitivity for SLN detection ranged from 50 to 100% with a pooled average of 86%.

The pitfalls of removing adipose tissue presuming as mapped lymph node leading to failure of SLNB as reported by Frumovitz et al[141] and challenges in SLNB from obesity can be subjugated with this technique.

Robert Holloway[142] combined blue dye with this technique and found 100% bilateral detection rates. When this technique was combined with Tc-99, similar detection rates were seen by How et al,[143] but better detection rates were shown by Togami et al.[144]

So, it can be concluded sentinel node mapping with a NIR imaging system with ICG dye with a robotic platform is highly effective, easy to master, and safe for sentinel node mapping. And the addition of combination methods to this technique may further improve the detection rates.

Learning Curve

Learning curve and surgeon's expertise are barriers to achieving high detection rates; this is reflected by low sensitivity noted in the pioneer study by Altgassen et al.[104] The proposed experience to gain proficiency for achieving a sufficient detection rate and acceptable false-negative rate of the technique is at least 20 to 30 procedures of SLNB, followed by systematic lymphadenectomy.[145]

Conclusion

Sentinel node appears as a promising diagnostic surgical approach in gynecological cancers to overcome disadvantages of systematic lymphadenectomy with added benefits; however, at present it has broad variations of acceptability in clinical practice of oncological surgeries. Increasing evidence of superior outcomes with the advanced technology of robotic platform along with fluoroprobes is opening doors to move forward in accepting SLNB as the standard of care in gynecological malignancies, especially endometrial cancer. However, irrespective of techniques, future research should look into limited evidence on oncological safety, quality of life, benefit, and treatment of increased detection of low-volume disease.

References

1. Gynecologic Oncology Group. Surgical procedures manual. Buffalo, NY: Gynecologic Oncology Group; 2007. Accessed April 2, 2012. http://www.gog.org
2. Mutch DN. The new FIGO staging system for cancers of the vulva, cervix, endometrium and sarcomas. Gynecol Oncol 2009;115:325–328

3. Benedetti Panici P, Basile S, Maneschi F, et al. Systematic pelvic lymphadenectomy vs. no lymphadenectomy in early-stage endometrial carcinoma: randomized clinical trial. J Natl Cancer Inst 2008;100(23):1707–1716

4. Kitchener H, Swart AM, Qian Q, Amos C, Parmar MK; ASTEC study group. Efficacy of systematic pelvic lymphadenectomy in endometrial cancer (MRC ASTEC trial): a randomised study. Lancet 2009;373(9658):125–136

5. Shah M, Lewin SN, Deutsch I, et al. Therapeutic role of lymphadenectomy for cervical cancer. Cancer 2011;117(2):310–317

6. Fuller AF Jr, Elliott N, Kosloff C, Hoskins WJ, Lewis JL Jr. Determinants of increased risk for recurrence in patients undergoing radical hysterectomy for stage IB and IIA carcinoma of the cervix. Gynecol Oncol 1989;33(1):34–39

7. Creutzberg CL, Lu KH, Fleming GF. Uterine cancer: adjuvant therapy and management of metastatic disease. J Clin Oncol 2019;37(27): 2490–2500

8. Dowdy SC, Borah BJ, Bakkum-Gamez JN, et al. Prospective assessment of survival, morbidity, and cost associated with lymphadenectomy in low-risk endometrial cancer. Gynecol Oncol 2012;127(1):5–10

9. Franchi M, Ghezzi F, Riva C, Miglierina M, Buttarelli M, Bolis P. Postoperative compli-cations after pelvic lymphadenectomy for the surgical staging of endometrial cancer. J Surg Oncol 2001;78(4):232–237, discussion 237–240

10. Matsuura Y, Kawagoe T, Toki N, Tanaka M, Kashimura M. Long-standing complications after treatment for cancer of the uterine cervix:clinical significance of medical examination at 5 years after treatment. Int J Gynecol Cancer 2006;16(1):294–297

11. Homesley HD, Kadar N, Barrett RJ, Lentz SS. Selective pelvic and periaortic lympha-denectomy does not increase morbidity in surgical staging of endometrial carcinoma. Am J Obstet Gynecol 1992;167(5):1225–1230

12. Cea García J, de la Riva Pérez PA, Rodríguez Jiménez I, et al. Selective biopsy of the sentinel node in cancer of cervix: experience in validation phase. Rev Esp Med Nucl Imagen Mol (Engl Ed) 2018;37(6):359–365

13. Gould EA, Winship T, Philbin PH, Kerr HH. Observations on a "sentinel node" in cancer of the parotid. Cancer 1960;13:77–78

14. Cabanas RM. An approach for the treatment of penile carcinoma. Cancer 1977;39(2):456–466

15. Morton DL, Wen DR, Wong JH, et al. Technical details of intraoperative lymphatic mapping for early stage melanoma. Arch Surg 1992; 127(4):392–399

16. Giuliano AE, Kirgan DM, Guenther JM, Morton DL. Lymphatic mapping and sentinel lymphadenectomy for breast cancer. Ann Surg 1994;220(3):391–398, discussion 398–401

17. Coit DG. Clinical Practice Guidelines in Oncology, Melanoma version 1. NCCN Guidelines Panel Members Melanoma; 2011

18. Carlson RW. NCCN Clinical Practice Guidelines in Oncology, Breast Cancer version 2. NCCN Guidelines Panel Members Breast Cancer; 2011

19. Levenback C, Burke TW, Gershenson DM, Morris M, Malpica A, Ross MI. Intraoperative lymphatic mapping for vulvar cancer. Obstet Gynecol 1994;84(2):163–167

20. Burke TW, Levenback C, Tornos C, Morris M, Wharton JT, Gershenson DM. Intraabdominal lymphatic mapping to direct selective pelvic and paraaortic lymphadenectomy in women with high-risk endometrial cancer: results of a pilot study. Gynecol Oncol 1996;62(2): 169–173

21. Echt ML, Finan MA, Hoffman MS, Kline RC, Roberts WS, Fiorica JV. Detection of sentinel lymph nodes with lymphazurin in cervical, uterine, and vulvar malignancies. South Med J 1999;92(2):204–208

22. Van der Zee AG, Oonk MH, De Hullu JA, et al. Sentinel node dissection is safe in the treatment of early-stage vulvar cancer. J Clin Oncol 2008;26(6):884–889.

23. Diaz JP, Gemignani ML, Pandit-Taskar N, et al. Sentinel lymph node biopsy in the management of early-stage cervical carcinoma. Gynecol Oncol 2011;120(3):347–352

24. Jakub JW, Pendas S, Reintgen DS. Current status of sentinel lymph node mapping and biopsy: facts and controversies. Oncologist 2003;8(1):59–68

25. Gortzak-Uzan L, Jimenez W, Nofech-Mozes S, et al. Sentinel lymph node biopsy vs. pelvic lymphadenectomy in early stage cervical cancer: is it time to change the gold standard? Gynecol Oncol 2010;116(1):28–32

26. Krag DN, Anderson SJ, Julian TB, et al. Sentinel-lymph-node resection compared with conventional axillary-lymph-node dissection in clinically node-negative patients with breast cancer: overall survival findings from the NSABP B-32 randomised phase 3 trial. Lancet Oncol 2010;11(10):927–933

27. Hauspy J, Verkinderen L, De Pooter C, Dirix LY, van Dam PA. Sentinel node metastasis in the groin detected by technetium-labeled

nannocolloid in a patient with cervical cancer. Gynecol Oncol 2002;86(3):358–360

28. Mathevet P. Surgical lymph-node evaluation in cervical cancer. Cancer Radiother 2009;13(6–7): 499–502

29. Horn LC, Hentschel B, Fischer U, Peter D, Bilek K. Detection of micrometastases in pelvic lymph nodes in patients with carcinoma of the cervix uteri using step sectioning: Frequency, topographic distribution and prognostic impact. Gynecol Oncol 2008;111(2):276–281

30. Holloway RW, Gupta S, Stavitzski NM, et al. Sentinel lymph node mapping with staging lymphadenectomy for patients with endometrial cancer increases the detection of metastasis. Gynecol Oncol 2016;141(2):206–210

31. Bats A-S, Buénerd A, Querleu D, et al; SENTICOL collaborative group. Diagnostic value of intraoperative examination of sentinel lymph node in early cervical cancer: a prospective, multicenter study. Gynecol Oncol 2011;123(2):230–235

32. Slama J, Dundr P, Dusek L, Cibula D. High false negative rate of frozen section examination of sentinel lymph nodes in patients with cervical cancer. Gynecol Oncol 2013;129(2):384–388

33. Holloway RW, Abu-Rustum NR, Backes FJ, et al. Sentinel lymph node mapping and staging in endometrial cancer: a Society of Gynecologic Oncology literature review with consensus recommendations. Gynecol Oncol 2017;146(2):405–415

34. Abu-Rustum NR, Khoury-Collado F, Pandit-Taskar N, et al. Sentinel lymph node mapping for grade 1 endometrial cancer: is it the answer to the surgical staging dilemma? Gynecol Oncol 2009;113(2):163–169

35. Ballester M, Dubernard G, Lécuru F, et al. Detection rate and diagnostic accuracy of sentinel-node biopsy in early stage endometrial cancer: a prospective multicentre study (SENTI-ENDO). Lancet Oncol 2011;12(5):469–476

36. Holman LL, Levenback CF, Frumovitz M. Sentinel lymph node evaluation in women with cervical cancer. J Minim Invasive Gynecol 2014;21(4):540–545

37. Papadia A, Gasparri ML, Buda A, Mueller MD. Sentinel lymph node mapping in endometrial cancer: comparison of fluorescence dye with traditional radiocolloid and blue. J Cancer Res Clin Oncol 2017;143(10):2039–2048

38. Nanocoll Ficha Técnica y Resúmen de las Características del Producto [Internet]. Ministerio de Sanidad, Política Social e Igualdad - Agencia Española de Medicamentos y Productos Sanitarios. https://www. aemps.

gob.es/cima/pdfs/es/ft/71080/   71080_ft.pdf [Accessed: August 13, 2017]

39. Dunnwald LK, Mankoff DA, Byrd DR, et al. Technical aspects of sentinel node lymphoscintigraphy for breast cancer. J Nucl Med Technol 1999;27(2):106–111 [] [Google Scholar]

40. Buda A, Elisei F, Dolci C, Cuzzocrea M, Milani R. Uterine lymphatic drainage is unaffected from injection technique and operators: Identical sentinel node detection in two cases of endometrial cancer. Int J Surg Case Rep 2013;4(8):697–699

41. Rocha A, Domínguez AM, Lécuru F, Bourdel N. Indocyanine green and infrared fluorescence in detection of sentinel lymph nodes in endometrial and cervical cancer staging: a systematic review. Eur J Obstet Gynecol Reprod Biol 2016;206:213–219

42. Darin MC, Gómez-Hidalgo NR, Westin SN, et al. Role of indocyanine green in sentinel node mapping in gynecologic cancer: is fluorescence imaging the new standard? J Minim Invasive Gynecol 2016;23(2):186–193

43. Surynt E, Reinholz-Jaskolska M, Bidzinski M. Laparoscopic sentinel lymph node mapping after cervical injection of indocyanine green for endometrial cancer: preliminary report. Wideochir Inne Tech Malo Inwazyjne 2015;10(3):406–412

44. Buda A, Crivellaro C, Elisei F, et al. Impact of indocyanine green for sentinel lymph node mapping in early stage endometrial and 28. cervical cancer: comparison with conventional radiotracer (99m)Tc and/or blue dye. Ann Surg Oncol 2016;23(7):2183–2191

45. Dargent D, Enria R. Laparoscopic assessment of the sentinel lymph nodes in early cervical cancer. Technique: preliminary results and future developments. Crit Rev Oncol Hematol 2003;48(3):305–310

46. Rossi EC, Ivanova A, Boggess JF. Robotically assisted fluorescence-guided lymph node mapping with ICG for gynecologic malignancies: a feasibility study. Gynecol Oncol 2012;124(1):78–82

47. Altgassen C, Müller N, Hornemann A, et al. Immunohistochemical workup of sentinel nodes in endometrial cancer improves diagnostic accuracy. Gynecol Oncol 2009; 114(2):284–287

48. Amoroso V, Generali D, Buchholz T, et al. International expert consensus on primary systemic therapy in the management of early breast cancer: Highlights of the Fifth Symposium on Primary Systemic Therapy in

the Management of Operable Breast Cancer, Cremona, Italy (2013). J Natl Cancer Inst Monogr 2015;2015(51):90–96

49. Cibula D, Abu-Rustum NR, Dusek L, et al. Bilateral ultrastaging of sentinel lymph node in cervical cancer: Lowering the false-negative rate and improving the detection of micrometastasis. Gynecol Oncol 2012; 127(3):462–466

50. Euscher ED, Malpica A, Atkinson EN, Levenback CF, Frumovitz M, Deavers MT. Ultrastaging improves detection of metastases in sentinel lymph nodes of uterine cervix squamous cell carcinoma. Am J Surg Pathol 2008;32(9): 1336–1343

51. Sartori E, Tisi G, Chiudinelli F, La Face B, Franzini R, Pecorelli S. Early stage cervical cancer: adjuvant treatment in negative lymph node cases. Gynecol Oncol 2007; 107(1, Suppl 1)S170–S174

52. Nagai T, Niikura H, Okamoto S, et al. A new diagnostic method for rapid detection of lymph node metastases using a one-step nucleic acid amplification (OSNA) assay in endometrial cancer. Ann Surg Oncol 2015;22(3):980–986

53. Todo Y, Kato H, Kaneuchi M, Watari H, Takeda M, Sakuragi N. Survival effect of para-aortic lymphadenectomy in endometrial cancer (SEPAL study): a retrospective cohort analysis. (Published erratum appears in *Lancet* 2010; 376: 594). Lancet 2010;375:1165–1172

54. Sharma C, Deutsch I, Lewin SN, et al. Lympha-denectomy influences the utilization of adjuvant radiation treatment for endometrial cancer. Am J Obstet Gynecol 2011;205(6):562. e1–562.e9

55. Hogberg T. Adjuvant chemotherapy in endometrial cancer. Int J Gynecol Cancer 2010; 20(11, Suppl 2)S57–S59

56. Burke WM, Orr J, Leitao M, et al; SGO Clinical Practice Endometrial Cancer Working Group; Society of Gynecologic Oncology Clinical Practice Committee. Endometrial cancer: a review and current management strategies: part II. Gynecol Oncol 2014;134(2):393–402

57. Burke WM, Orr J, Leitao M, et al; SGO Clinical Practice Endometrial Cancer Working Group; Society of Gynecologic Oncology Clinical Practice Committee. Endometrial cancer: a review and current management strategies: part I. Gynecol Oncol 2014;134(2):385–392

58. Abu-Rustum NR. Sentinel lymph node mapping for endometrial cancer: a modern approach to surgical staging. J Natl Compr Canc Netw 2014;12(2):288–297

59. Fayna Ferkle N, Nicole McMillian P, Jillian Scavone M, et al. NCCN guidelines index uterine neoplasms TOC discussion NCCN guidelines, version 2. 2016 panel members uterine neoplasms MD/liaison, Dana-Farber/ Brigham and Women's Cancer Center. https:// www.nccn.org/professionals/physician_gls/ pdf/ uterine.pdf. [Accessed May 30, 2016]

60. Ruscito I, Gasparri ML, Braicu EI, et al. Sentinel node mapping in cervical and endo-metrial cancer: indocyanine green versus other conventional dyes—a meta-analysis. Ann Surg Oncol 2016;23(11):3749–3756

61. Xiong L, Gazyakan E, Yang W, et al. Indocyanine green fluorescence-guided sentinel node biopsy: a meta-analysis on detection rate and diagnostic performance. Eur J Surg Oncol 2014;40(7):843–849

62. Khoury-Collado F, Abu-Rustum NR. Lymphatic mapping in endometrial cancer: a literature review of current techniques and results. Int J Gynecol Cancer 2008;18(6):1163–1168

63. Kang S, Yoo HJ, Hwang JH, Lim MC, Seo SS, Park SY. Sentinel lymph node biopsy in endometrial cancer: meta-analysis of 26 studies. Gynecol Oncol 2011;123(3):522–527

64. Mariani A, Dowdy SC, Cliby WA, et al. Prospective assessment of lymphatic dissemination in endometrial cancer: a paradigm shift in surgical staging. Gynecol Oncol. 2008;109(1):11–18

65. Mariani A, Dowdy SC, Cliby WA, et al. Prospective assessment of lymphatic dissemination in endometrial cancer: a paradigm shift in surgical staging. Gynecol Oncol 2008;109(1):11–18

66. Holloway RW, Ahmad S, Kendrick JE, et al. A prospective cohort study comparing colorimetric and fluorescent imaging for sentinel lymph node mapping in endometrial cancer. Ann Surg Oncol 2017;24(7):1972–1979

67. Mariani A, Dowdy SC, Cliby WA, et al. Prospective assessment of lymphatic dissemination in endometrial cancer: a paradigm shift in surgical staging. Gynecol Oncol 2008;109(1):11–18

68. Abu-Rustum NR, Gomez JD, Alektiar KM, et al. The incidence of isolated paraaortic nodal metastasis in surgically staged endometrial cancer patients with negative pelvic lymph nodes. Gynecol Oncol 2009;115(2):236–238

69. Milam MR, Java J, Walker JL, Metzinger DS, Parker LP, Coleman RL; Gynecologic Oncology Group. Nodal metastasis risk in endometrioid endometrial cancer. Obstet Gynecol 2012;119(2 Pt 1):286–292

70. Gala RB, Margulies R, Steinberg A, et al; Society of Gynecologic Surgeons Systematic Review

Group. Systematic review of robotic surgery in gynecology: robotic techniques compared with laparoscopy and laparotomy. J Minim Invasive Gynecol 2014;21(3):353–361

71. Gehrig PA, Cantrell LA, Shafer A, Abaid LN, Mendivil A, Boggess JF. What is the optimal minimally invasive surgical procedure for endometrial cancer staging in the obese and morbidly obese woman? Gynecol Oncol 2008;111(1):41–45

72. Rossi EC, Kowalski LD, Scalici J, et al. A comparison of sentinel lymph node biopsy to lymphadenectomy for endometrial cancer staging (FIRES trial): a multicentre, prospective, cohort study. Lancet Oncol 2017;18(3):384–392.28159465

73. Bodurtha Smith AJ, Fader AN, Tanner EJ. Sentinel lymph node assessment in endometrial cancer: a systematic review and meta-analysis. Am J Obstet Gynecol 2017;216(5):459–476.e10

74. Barlin JN, Khoury-Collado F, Kim CH, et al. The importance of applying a sentinel lymph node mapping algorithm in endometrial cancer staging: beyond removal of blue nodes. Gynecol Oncol 2012;125(3):531–535

75. Mais V, Peiretti M, Gargiulo T, Parodo G, Cirronis MG, Melis GB. Intraoperative sentinel lymph node detection by vital dye through laparoscopy or laparotomy in early endometrial cancer. J Surg Oncol 2010;101(5):408–412

76. Piver MS, Rutledge F, Smith JP. Five classes of extended hysterectomy for women with cervical cancer. Obstet Gynecol 1974;44(2):265–272

77. Landoni F, Maneo A, Cormio G, et al. Class II versus class III radical hysterectomy in stage IB-IIA cervical cancer: a prospective randomized study. Gynecol Oncol 2001;80(1):3–12

78. Diaz JP, Sonoda Y, Leitao MM Jr, et al. Oncologic outcome of fertility-sparing radical trachelectomy versus radical hysterectomy for stage IB1 cervical carcinoma. Gynecol Oncol 2008;111(2):255–260

79. Creasman WT, Kohler MF. Is lymph vascular space involvement an independent prognostic factor in early cervical cancer? Gynecol Oncol 2004;92(2):525–529

80. Delgado G, Bundy B, Zaino R, Sevin BU, Creasman WT, Major F. Prospective surgical-pathological study of disease-free interval in patients with stage IB squamous cell carcinoma of the cervix: a Gynecologic Oncology Group study. Gynecol Oncol 1990;38(3):352–357

81. Yuan C, Wang P, Lai C, Tsu E, Yen M, Ng H. Recurrence and survival analyses of

1,115 cervical cancer patients treated with radical hysterectomy. Gynecol Obstet Invest 1999;47(2):127–132

82. Biewenga P, van der Velden J, Mol BW, et al. Prognostic model for survival in patients with early stage cervical cancer. Cancer 2011;117(4):768–776

83. Wolfson AH, Varia MA, Moore D, et al; American College of Radiology (ACR). ACR Appropriateness Criteria® role of adjuvant therapy in the management of early stage cervical cancer. Gynecol Oncol 2012;125(1):256–262

84. Bhatla N, Berek JS, Cuello Fredes M, et al. Revised FIGO staging for carcinoma of the cervix uteri. Int J Gynaecol Obstet 2019;145(1):129–145

85. Delgado G, Bundy BN, Fowler WC Jr, et al. A prospective surgical pathological study of stage I squamous carcinoma of the cervix: a Gynecologic Oncology Group Study. Gynecol Oncol 1989;35(3):314–320

86. Look KY, Brunetto VL, Clarke-Pearson DL, et al. An analysis of cell type in patients with surgically staged stage IB carcinoma of the cervix: a Gynecologic Oncology Group study. Gynecol Oncol 1996;63(3):304–311

87. Magrina JF, Goodrich MA, Lidner TK, Weaver AL, Cornella JL, Podratz KC. Modified radical hysterectomy in the treatment of early squamous cervical cancer. Gynecol Oncol 1999;72(2):183–186

88. Di Stefano AB, Acquaviva G, Garozzo G, et al. Lymph node mapping and sentinel node detection in patients with cervical carcinoma: a 2-year experience. Gynecol Oncol 2005;99(3):671–679

89. Leveuf J, Godard H. Les lymphatique de l'uterus. Rev Chir 1923;3:219–248

90. Abu-Rustum NR, Khoury-Collado F, Gemignani ML. Techniques of sentinel lymph node identification for early-stage cervical and uterine cancer. Gynecol Oncol 2008; 111(2, suppl)S44–S50

91. Schwendinger V, Müller-Holzner E, Zeimet AG, Marth C. Sentinel node detection with the blue dye technique in early cervical cancer. Eur J Gynaecol Oncol 2006;27(4):359–362

92. O'Boyle JD, Coleman RL, Bernstein SG, Lifshitz S, Muller CY, Miller DS. Intraoperative lymphatic mapping in cervix cancer patients undergoing radical hysterectomy: A pilot study. Gynecol Oncol 2000;79(2):238–243

93. Marchiolè P, Buénerd A, Scoazec JY, Dargent D, Mathevet P. Sentinel lymph node biopsy is

not accurate in predicting lymph node status for patients with cervical carcinoma. Cancer 2004;100(10):2154–2159

94. Du XL, Sheng XG, Jiang T, et al. Sentinel lymph node biopsy as guidance for radical trachelectomy in young patients with early stage cervical cancer. BMC Cancer 2011;11:157

95. Ogawa S, Kobayashi H, Amada S, et al. Sentinel node detection with (99m)Tc phytate alone is satisfactory for cervical cancer patients undergoing radical hysterectomy and pelvic lymphadenectomy. Int J Clin Oncol 2010; 15(1):52–58

96. Darlin L, Persson J, Bossmar T, et al. The sentinel node concept in early cervical cancer performs well in tumors smaller than 2 cm. Gynecol Oncol 2010;117(2):266–269

97. Lécuru F, Mathevet P, Querleu D, et al. Bilateral negative sentinel nodes accurately predict absence of lymph node metastasis in early cervical cancer: results of the SENTICOL study. J Clin Oncol 2011;29(13):1686–1691; E-pub ahead of print

98. Plante M, Renaud MC, Têtu B, Harel F, Roy M. Laparoscopic sentinel node mapping in early-stage cervical cancer. Gynecol Oncol 2003;91(3):494–503

99. Niikura H, Okamura C, Akahira J, et al. Sentinel lymph node detection in early cervical cancer with combination 99mTc phytate and patent blue. Gynecol Oncol 2004;94(2):528–532

100. van de Lande J, Torrenga B, Raijmakers PG, et al. Sentinel lymph node detection in early stage uterine cervix carcinoma: a systematic review. Gynecol Oncol 2007;106(3):604–613

101. Pandit-Taskar N, Gemignani ML, Lyall A, Larson SM, Barakat RR, Abu Rustum NR. Single photon emission computed tomography SPECT-CT improves sentinel node detection and localization in cervical and uterine malignancy. Gynecol Oncol 2010;117(1):59–64

102. Kraft O, Havel M. Detection of sentinel lymph nodes in gynecologic tumours by planar scintigraphy and SPECT/CT. Mol Imaging Radionucl Ther 2012;21(2):47–55

103. Díaz-Feijoo B, Pérez-Benavente MA, Cabrera-Diaz S, et al. Change in clinical management of sentinel lymph node location in early stage cervical cancer: the role of SPECT/CT. Gynecol Oncol 2011;120(3):353–357

104. Altgassen C, Hertel H, Brandstädt A, Köhler C, Dürst M, Schneider A; AGO Study Group. Multicenter validation study of the sentinel lymph node concept in cervical cancer: AGO Study Group. J Clin Oncol 2008;26(18): 2943–2951

105. Medl M, Peters-Engl C, Schütz P, Vesely M, Sevelda P. First report of lymphatic mapping with isosulfan blue dye and sentinel node biopsy in cervical cancer. Anticancer Res 2000;20(2B):1133–1134

106. Juretzka MM, Jensen KC, Longacre TA, Teng NN, Husain A. Detection of pelvic lymph node micrometastasis in stage IA2-IB2 cervical cancer by immunohistochemical analysis. Gynecol Oncol 2004;93(1):107–111

107. Fregnani JH, Latorre MR, Novik PR, Lopes A, Soares FA. Assessment of pelvic lymph node micrometastatic disease in stages IB and IIA of carcinoma of the uterine cervix. Int J Gynecol Cancer 2006;16(3):1188–1194

108. Marchiolé P, Buénerd A, Benchaib M, Nezhat K, Dargent D, Mathevet P. Clinical significance of lympho vascular space involvement and lymph node micrometastases in early-stage cervical cancer: a retrospective case-control surgico-pathological study. Gynecol Oncol 2005;97(3):727–732

109. Sonoda K, Yahata H, Okugawa K, et al. Value of intraoperative cytological and pathological sentinel lymph node diagnosis in fertility-sparing trachelectomy for early-stage cervical cancer. Oncology 2018;94(2):92–98

110. Levenback C, Coleman RL, Burke TW, et al. Lymphatic mapping and sentinel node identification in patients with cervix cancer undergoing radical hysterectomy and pelvic lymphadenectomy. J Clin Oncol 2002;20(3): 688–693

111. Rob L, Strnad P, Robova H, et al. Study of lymphatic mapping and sentinel node identification in early stage cervical cancer. Gynecol Oncol 2005;98(2):281–288

112. Cormier B, Diaz JP, Shih K, et al. Establishing a sentinel lymph node mapping algorithm for the treatment of early cervical cancer. Gynecol Oncol 2011;122(2):275–280

113. Eiriksson LR, Covens A. Sentinel lymph node mapping in cervical cancer: the future? BJOG 2012;119(2):129–133

114. Covens A, Rosen B, Murphy J, et al. How important is removal of the parametrium at surgery for carcinoma of the cervix? Gynecol Oncol 2002;84(1):145–149

115. Dostalek L, Åvall-Lundqvist E, Creutzberg CL, et al. ESGO survey on current practice in the management of cervical cancer. Int J Gynecol Cancer 2018;28(6):1226–1231

116. NCC Network, Others. NCCN clinical practice guidelines in oncology (NCCN guidelines): cervical cancer. Version 1. 2016, 2016

117. Alkatout I, Schubert M, Garbrecht N, et al. Vulvar cancer: epidemiology, clinical presentation, and management options. Int J Womens Health 2015;7:305–313

118. Homesley HD, Bundy BN, Sedlis A, et al. Assessment of current International Federation of Gynecology and Obstetrics staging of vulvar carcinoma relative to prognostic factors for survival (a Gynecologic Oncology Group study). Am J Obstet Gynecol 1991;164(4):997–1003, discussion 1003–1004

119. Hacker NF, Leuchter RS, Berek JS, Castaldo TW, Lagasse LD. Radical vulvectomy and bilateral inguinal lymphadenectomy through separate groin incisions. Obstet Gynecol 1981;58(5):574–579

120. Bell JG, Lea JS, Reid GC. Complete groin lymphadenectomy with preservation of the fascia lata in the treatment of vulvar carcinoma. Gynecol Oncol 2000;77(2):314–318

121. Johann S, Klaeser B, Krause T, Mueller MD. Comparison of outcome and recurrence-free survival after sentinel lymph node biopsy and lymphadenectomy in vulvar cancer. Gynecol Oncol 2008;110(3):324–328

122. Farrell R, Gebski V, Hacker NF. Quality of life after complete lymphadenectomy for vulvar cancer: do women prefer sentinel lymph node biopsy? Int J Gynecol Cancer 2014;24(4):813–819

123. Van der Zee AGJ, Oonk MH, De Hullu JA, et al. Sentinel node dissection is safe in the treatment of early-stage vulvar cancer. J Clin Oncol 2008;26(6):884–889

124. Levenback CF, Ali S, Coleman RL, et al. Lymphatic mapping and sentinel lymph node biopsy in women with squamous cell carcinoma of the vulva: a gynecologic oncology group study. J Clin Oncol 2012;30(31):3786–3791

125. Greer BE, Koh WJ. New NCCN guidelines for vulvar cancer. J Natl Compr Canc Netw 2016;14(5, Suppl)656–658

126. Covens A, Vella ET, Kennedy EB, Reade CJ, Jimenez W, Le T. Sentinel lymph node biopsy in vulvar cancer: systematic review, meta-analysis and guideline recommendations. Gynecol Oncol 2015;137(2):351–361

127. Robison K, Fiascone S, Moore R. Vulvar cancer and sentinel lymph nodes: a new standard of care? Expert Rev Anticancer Ther 2014;14(9):975–977

128. Belhocine TZ, Prefontaine M, Lanvin D, et al. Added-value of SPECT/CT to lymphatic mapping and sentinel lymphadenectomy in gynaecological cancers. Am J Nucl Med Mol Imaging 2013;3(2):182–193

129. Mohammad A, Hunter MI. Robot-assisted sentinel lymph node mapping and inguinal lymph node dissection using near-infrared fluorescence in vulvar cancer. J Minim Invasive Gynecol 2019;26(5):968–972

130. Frumovitz M, Gayed IW, Jhingran A, et al. Lymphatic mapping and sentinel lymph node detection in women with vaginal cancer. Gynecol Oncol 2008;108(3):478–481

131. Ayhan A, Celik H, Dursun P. Lymphatic mapping and sentinel node biopsy in gynecological cancers: a critical review of the literature. World J Surg Oncol 2008;6:53

132. Hertel H, Soergel P, Muecke J, et al. Is there a place for sentinel technique in treatment of vaginal cancer? Feasibility, clinical experience, and results. Int J Gynecol Cancer 2013;23(9):1692–1698

133. Kobayashi K, Ramirez PT, Kim EE, et al. Sentinel node mapping in vulvovaginal melanoma using SPECT/CT lymphoscintigraphy. Clin Nucl Med 2009;34(12):859–861

134. Kleppe M, Brans B, Van Gorp T, et al. The detection of sentinel nodes in ovarian cancer: a feasibility study. J Nucl Med 2014;55(11):1799–1804

135. Lago V, Bello P, Montero B, et al. Clinical application of the sentinel lymph node technique in early ovarian cancer: a pilot study. Int J Gynecol Cancer 2019;29(2):377–381

136. El-Ghobashy AE, Saidi SA. Sentinel lymph node sampling in gynaecological cancers: techniques and clinical applications. Eur J Surg Oncol 2009;35(7):675–685

137. Hassanzadeh M, Hosseini Farahabadi E, Yousefi Z, Kadkhodayan S, Zarifmahmoudi L, Sadeghi R. Lymphatic mapping and sentinel node biopsy in ovarian tumors: a study using intra-operative Tc-99m-Phytate and lymphoscintigraphy imaging. J Ovarian Res 2016;9(1):55

138. Frey MK, Ihnow SB, Worley MJ Jr, et al. Minimally invasive staging of endometrial cancer is feasible and safe in elderly women. J Minim Invasive Gynecol 2011;18(2):200–204

139. Rajanbabu A, Murali V, Nataraj YS, Vijaykumar DK. Detection of sentinel lymph nodes in endometrial cancer with intracervical indocyanine green injection and robotically assisted near infrared imaging: a feasibility study in Indian setting. Indian J Gynecol Oncolog 2015;13:1–6

140. Wu Y, Jing J, Wang J, Xu B, Du M, Chen M. Robotic-assisted sentinel lymph node mapping with indocyanine green in pelvic

malignancies: a systematic review and meta-analysis. Front Oncol 2019;9:585

141. Frumovitz M, Plante M, Lee PS, et al. Near-infrared fluorescence for detection of sentinel lymph nodes in women with cervical and uterine cancers (FILM): a randomised, phase 3, multicentre, non-inferiority trial. Lancet Oncol 2018;19(10):1394–1403

142. Holloway RW, Bravo RA, Rakowski JA, et al. Detection of sentinel lymph nodes in patients with endometrial cancer undergoing robotic-assisted staging: a comparison of colorimetric and fluorescence imaging. Gynecol Oncol 2012;126(1):25–29

143. How J, Gotlieb WH, Press JZ, et al. Comparing indocyanine green, technetium, and blue dye for sentinel lymph node mapping in endometrial cancer. Gynecol Oncol 2015;137(3): 436–442

144. Togami S, Kawamura T, Fukuda M, Yanazume S, Kamio M, Kobayashi H. Prospective study of sentinel lymph node mapping for endometrial cancer. Int J Gynaecol Obstet 2018;143(3): 313–318

145. Khoury-Collado F, Glaser GE, Zivanovic O, et al. Improving sentinel lymph node detection rates in endometrial cancer: how many cases are needed? Gynecol Oncol 2009;115(3):453–455

Accompanying Video

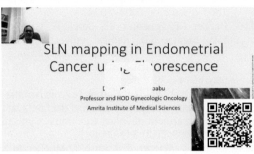

Video 9.1   SLN and ICG. https://www.thieme.de/de/q.htm?p=opn/cs/21/6/15245409-7631da67

10 Robotic Pelvic and Para-aortic Lymph Node Dissection

Somashekhar S.P. and Priya Kapoor

Introduction

Lymphatics are an essential pathway for spread and are prognostic indicators in gynecologic malignancies, so appropriate management of pelvic and para-aortic lymph nodes is a crucial component of treatment. The intent of pelvic and para-aortic lymphadenectomy can be diagnostic or therapeutic and has been extensively studied but is controversial. Over the past few decades, laparotomy has been replaced by minimally invasive techniques and robotic surgery has unquestionably alchemized surgical staging in early gynecologic malignancies. Retroperitoneal lymph nodes in cervical, endometrial, and even ovarian malignancies have been successfully addressed by robotic surgery.

This chapter deals with robotic surgical technology in pelvic and para-aortic lymphadenectomy, addressing the techniques and tips most helpful in performing a safe and complete robotic pelvic and para-aortic lymphadenectomy.

Indications of Pelvic and Para-aortic Lymph Node Dissection in Gynecologic Malignancies

The role of lymphadenectomy in gynecologic malignancies is controversial, whether it is a therapeutic procedure or staging.

Here the benefits of pelvic and para-aortic lymphadenectomy can be analyzed in two ways:

1. **In advanced cases:** Direct survival benefit following therapeutic lymphadenectomy of bulky positive metastatic lymph nodes.[1]

2. **In early disease:** Indirect survival benefits from systematic lymphadenectomy, giving accurate staging of the disease and helps in planning tailor-made adjuvant treatment.[1]

It is largely accepted that in early ovarian, uterine, and cervical malignancy, lymphadenectomy is a good staging protocol and changes management.

In advanced gynecologic malignancies, debulking has emerging evidence, but its role in improving overall survival needs further trials.

The indication and controversies regarding pelvic and para-aortic lymphadenectomy in various gynecologic malignancies are discussed below.

Endometrial Cancer

Despite the shift to surgical staging by FIGO for improvements in staging accuracy, controversies continue regarding the benefits and extent of routine systematic pelvic and aortic lymphadenectomy, particularly in women presumed to have the early disease.

In 1987, the Gynecologic Oncology Group 33 study described the increased risk for pelvic lymph node metastasis in endometrial cancers (ECs) with deep myometrial invasion and higher grade. Hence complete lymph node dissection (LND) was considered to be reasonable for both therapeutic and prognostic benefit.[2] Owing to the added lower extremity lymphedema associated with this approach, the routine complete pelvic and para-aortic LND was challenged by the publication of two randomized trials.

Evidence Against Routine Lymphadenectomy

In the trial by Benedetti Panici and A Study in the Treatment of Endometrial Cancer (ASTEC) trial, systematic LND showed no difference in overall survival. These trials demonstrated that systemic LND did not offer a survival advantage in women with EC.[3,4] Several critiques of these results with study design and quality of surgery prompted many surgeons to disregard the data.

Evidence Supporting Lymphadenectomy

In contrast, Todo et al[5] published that patients with high-risk histologies or deep invasion who underwent para-aortic and pelvic lymphadenectomy had improved overall survival compared to patients with pelvic lymphadenectomy alone (HR 0.53; 95% CI 0.38–0.76, p < 0.001).

However, well-designed studies to answer this are lacking, and gaps remain in the definitive data regarding the role of lymphadenectomy in EC. The approach to lymph node evaluation in women with EC is debated, and practice varies across different institutions or surgeons.

Extent of Lymphadenectomy

Routine complete bilateral pelvic and aortic LND accurately determines the extent of malignancy to plan tailor-made adjuvant therapy. But the prime concern with regards to its universal use is the morbidity of lower extremity lymphedema and associated cellulitis.

Due to the lack of evidence of a therapeutic benefit of LND, less invasive techniques like sentinel lymph node (SLN) have become standard management of EC and have replaced complete lymphadenectomy or no lymphadenectomy in women with apparently uterine-confined EC.

Complete pelvic lymphadenectomy: The reported risk of lymphedema varies widely (5–38%).[6,7] Factors associated with lymphedema included advancing age, more than eight lymph nodes removed, obesity, and radiation therapy. Lymphedema was associated with clinically significant reductions in the quality-of-life domain.

Aortic lymph node dissection: The extent of LND, that is, whether para-aortic lymph nodes should be addressed and to what anatomic level

is also a matter of debate. The decision to dissect the aortic lymph nodes in EC is based on data suggesting that the risk for aortic metastasis increases in the presence of pelvic lymph node metastasis,[8,9] that isolated aortic lymph node recurrences occur,[9] and that survival is improved when aortic LND is included with pelvic LND.[5] Identifying patients at lower risk for aortic metastasis has led to many surgeons omitting aortic LND when the risk of metastasis is predicted to be lower than the procedure to remove the lymph nodes.

A prospective series reported that 77% of patients with para-aortic nodal metastases have disease above the inferior mesenteric artery.[10] Hence, the experts recommend extending the para-aortic LND superiorly to the level of the renal veins.

Selective Lymphadenectomy

In this approach, LND is performed only in patients with a higher risk for lymph node metastasis. There is no unanimity or defined criteria of "high-risk" patients, but the following factors are associated with an increased probability of retroperitoneal lymph node metastasis:

- Grade 3 endometrioid ECs and the nonendometrioid histologies: serous, clear cell, mixed cell, and undifferentiated.
- Tumors with deep invasion with one-half or more of the myometrium on preoperative imaging or intraoperative assessment.
- Large tumors >2 cm on preoperative imaging or intraoperative evaluation.

MAYO Criteria

The above criteria is based on a study of 328 patients forming the *"Mayo criteria"* that found that patients with EC with grade 1 to 2 endometrioid histology, tumor size of 2 cm or less, and 50% or less myometrial invasion (clinically or on the frozen section) have a 5% or lower chance of nodal metastasis, and thus, it is reasonable to omit LND in this population.[11]

Large prospective datasets have also validated these factors as predictive markers for lymph node metastasis.[10,12] These studies have shown that in the absence of these factors, the risk of retroperitoneal lymph node metastasis is approximately 1%.[13]

Similarly, in cases undergoing pelvic LND, aortic LND may be omitted in patients with low-grade disease, with <50% myometrial invasion, and without clinical evidence of pelvic lymph node metastases.[14]

A limitation of selective LND is the reliance on intraoperative frozen sections.

- In the authors' practice, all patients of EC undergo SLN, and the high-risk patients defined below are taken up for para-aortic lymphadenectomy.
  - FIGO grade 3.
  - Tumor >2 cm.
  - Pelvic node positive and >50% myome trial invasion.
  - Systematic PLND and para-aortic node dissection is performed up to renal veins.

Cervical Cancer

Pelvic and para-aortic lymphadenectomy procedures are performed for cervical cancer in the following clinical settings:

- Lymphadenectomy is a necessary part of radical hysterectomy for early stage cervical cancer and was first described by Wertheim in 1898.
- In addition, lymph node sampling is performed in some women treated with primary chemoradiation.
- In the advanced-stage disease, aortic lymphadenectomy may be performed either to remove known bulky metastasis prior to definitive radiation therapy or to stage patients with normal-appearing lymph nodes to tailor-make the extent of the radiotherapy fields.

A study by Gold MA showed that surgical exclusion compared with the radiographic exclusion of positive PALNs in patients with cervical cancer who received chemoradiation (RT plus C-based chemotherapy) had a significant prognostic impact.[15]

SLN biopsy is currently investigational.[16,17]

Lymph Node Dissection

LND debulks enlarged nodes, which leads to a therapeutic benefit and provides adequate staging information for treatment planning to individualize the radiotherapy field.[18]

The necessity for and extent of lymphadenectomy (pelvic, para-aortic) depends upon disease stage and imaging findings:

Stage IA1 squamous cell cervical cancer: The risk of lymph node metastases is 1% or less and lymphadenectomy is not performed unless there is lymphovascular space invasion, which is also rarely encountered at this early stage.[19] This is for both squamous cell carcinoma and adenocarcinoma.[20]

- **Stage IA2 disease or microscopic IB1 disease:** (nonvisible, >5 mm in depth and ≤4 cm in greatest dimension), the risk of nodal metastasis is 2 to 8%, and pelvic lymphadenectomy alone is generally sufficient since the risk for para-aortic nodal metastases is quite small.[6,19]

However, if pretreatment imaging shows positive or suspicious para-aortic nodes or if enlarged or fixed pelvic nodes are encountered during surgery, frozen section should be performed. If metastases are confirmed, we abandon the surgery and subject the patient to definitive chemoradiation; para-aortic lymphadenectomy should be completed as well in suspicious/enlarged nodes.

- **Macroscopic Stage IB1 and IIA1 tumors:** A complete pelvic lymphadenectomy should be performed at the time of hysterectomy. Para-aortic lymphadenectomy is performed at the surgeon's discretion and when pelvic lymph nodes are enlarged or fixed. Para-aortic lymphadenectomy is performed at the surgeon's discretion or when:
  - Pretreatment imaging demonstrates para-aortic nodes suspicious for metastatic disease.
  - Enlarged or fixed pelvic lymph nodes are encountered at surgery.
  - Frozen section of the pelvic nodes is positive, and metastases are confirmed.

Several trials have identified that bulky pelvic and/or para-aortic nodes (>2 cm) are resistant to radiotherapy and/or chemotherapy, and they pose a serious challenge.[21,22] Hence, surgical debulking of enlarged lymph nodes would be effective in chemoradiation-resistant lymph nodes.

The study by Moore KN presented an extra-peritoneal method for removing the pelvic and para-aortic lymph nodes with acceptable complications and no significant delay in initiating chemoradiation. It showed that an accurate assessment of lymphatic metastases resulted in modification of the radiation field, which, along with surgical debulking, improved overall survival.[23]

Sentinel Lymph Node Biopsy

Sentinel lymph node biopsy (SLNB) for patients with cervical cancer appears promising and is a National Comprehensive Cancer Network (NCCN)-approved option for those surgeons experienced with the procedure.[24,25] Four criteria are widely accepted as necessary for determining which patients should undergo SLNB and include:

- Tumors <4 cm.
- No suspicious lymph nodes are identified during preoperative imaging.
- Bilateral SLN detection.
- Ultrastaging (i.e., enhanced pathologic review, including additional sectioning and staining of the SLN).

Ovarian Cancer

Seventy-five percent of patients are diagnosed with ovarian cancer, unfortunately, stages II or higher. In this subset of patients, the role of lymphadenectomy has less prognostic and treatment planning implications than that for the patients with ovary-confined disease. However, it is essential to remove all suspicious and grossly enlarged nodes in patients with advanced disease to optimal cytoreductive surgery.[26,27] Burghardt et al compared complete pelvic lymphadenectomy or pelvic and para-aortic lymphadenectomy in 180 ovarian cancer patients with stage I to IV. The incidence of positive lymph nodes was 24% in stage I, 50% in stage II, 74% in stage III, and 73% in stage IV.[28] Some data suggest that LND is therapeutic in a portion of patients with advanced-stage disease.[29,30,31,32] However, the LION trial, a randomized phase III trial, concluded no additional benefit of lymphadenectomy in the absence of suspicious lymph nodes and otherwise completely resected advanced ovarian cancer.[33]

Evidence for Minimally Invasive Pelvic and Para-aortic Lymph Node Dissection

Randomized trials LAP2[34] and LACE[35] have validated that minimally invasive approaches in pelvic and para-aortic lymphadenectomy result in lower rates of peri- and postoperative complications as compared to open approach, without compromising the oncologic outcomes.

- Robotic surgery: There is evidence that robotic surgery is associated with similar short-term outcomes, shorter operating room time, and lower conversion rates to laparotomy than conventional laparoscopic surgery. In obese patients, robotic hysterectomy may reduce conversions because of positional intolerance.[36]
  - A randomized trial by Mäenpää et al ($n = 99$) of robotic versus laparoscopic staging for EC found shorter operative duration for robotic group (139 min vs. 170 min).[37] There were no conversions to laparotomy in the robotic group compared with 5 of 49 cases in the laparoscopy group. There were no differences in the number of lymph nodes removed, bleeding, or the length of postoperative hospital stay.
  - A database study including 1027 women with EC who underwent laparoscopic hysterectomy and 1437 who underwent robotic hysterectomy also found no difference in rate of complications with robotic compared with laparoscopic surgery.[38]
  - Study by Somashekhar et al[39] comparing robotic-assisted surgery and open surgery for high-risk EC in terms of systematic high para-aortic lymphadenectomy has the same oncological outcomes, as far as the completeness of systematic surgical staging is concerned; in addition, robotic surgery showed all the advantages of minimally

invasive technique and benefits to the patient. The study concluded:

○ LND is not inferior to the open method.

○ Blood loss, hospital stay, and pain were less.

○ Quicker recovery and early return to normal activities.

○ Smaller incision and improved cosmesis.

○ Better clinical outcome and patient's satisfaction.

Robotic Pelvic and Para-aortic Lymph Node Dissection

It has been established that[40] lymphatics in the uterine corpus drain primarily into the iliac lymph nodes. In the fundus region, the lymphatics may travel with the ovarian vessels directly to the para-aortic lymph nodes. Other pathways may also lead to the hypogastric or common iliac lymph nodes (**Fig. 10.1**).

Lymphadenectomy is an essential part of any oncological surgery more so with gynecologic malignancies. The lymphatics always follow the venous distribution and the point at which they drop into the major vessels lymphatic splash occurs and that is the most common site of tumor deposits. So accordingly in uterine malignancy,

through the internal iliac artery and vein obturator, parametrial and iliac nodal spread is common. Whereas in uterine fundal and ovarian tumors through the infundibulopelvic ligament, it drains into para-aortic lymph nodes.

On the right side, the infundibulopelvic (IP) ligament drains into inferior vena cava (IVC) one inch below the renal vein, so the retrocaval and paracaval nodes below the IVC are most commonly involved.

On the left side, the IP ligament drains into the left renal vein, leading to the fork node being most commonly involved.

Para-aortic is divided into two compartments—above and below the inferior mesenteric artery.

The lymph node classification, according to Benedetti-Panici et al includes eight pelvic and eight aortic groups.

The *pelvic groups* are external iliac, superficial obturator, deep obturator, common iliac, superficial internal iliac, deep internal iliac, presacral, and parametrial.

The *aortic groups* are precaval, paracaval, superficial intercavoaortic, deep intercavoaortic, preaortic, para-aortic, retrocaval, and retroaortic.

Pelvic Lymphadenectomy

According to the Gynecologic Oncology Group Surgical Procedures Manual, pelvic node dissection includes bilateral removal of nodal tissue

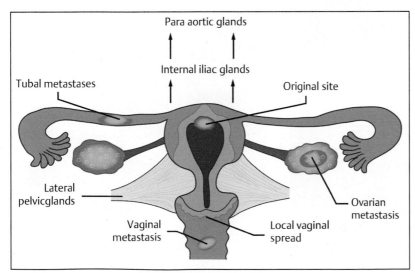

Para aortic glands

Internal iliac glands

Tubal metastases

Original site

Lateral pelvicglands

Ovarian metastasis

Vaginal metastasis

Local vaginal spread

Fig. 10.1 Anatomical considerations of boundaries of dissection.

from the distal half of each common iliac artery, the anterior and medial aspect of the proximal half of the external iliac artery and vein, and the distal half of the obturator fat pad anterior to the obturator nerve.[41] Most of the pelvic lymph nodes lie anterior, medially, and posteriorly to the external and internal iliac vessels and the obturator nerve. There are a few nodes that lie lateral to these structures, between the vessels and the pelvic sidewall, and these are generally removed in a complete dissection.[42]

The anatomical boundaries are:

- Anatomical spaces in pelvic dissection:
  - Paravesical space.
  - Pararectal space.

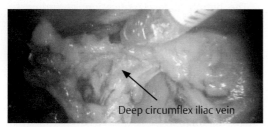

Fig. 10.2   Pelvic lymphadenectomy: Distal boundary.

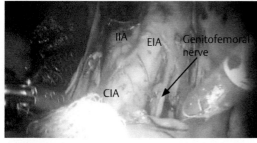

Fig. 10.3   Pelvic lymphadenectomy: Lateral and proximal boundary.

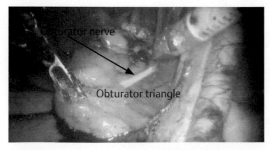

Fig. 10.4   Pelvic lymphadenectomy: Inferior boundary.

- Anatomical boundaries (**Figs. 10.2, 10.3** and **10.4**):
  - Distal: Deep circumflex iliac vein.
  - Proximal: Common iliac vessels.
  - Laterally: Genitofemoral nerve.
  - Inferiorly: Obturator fossa.

Para-aortic Lymph Node Dissection

According to the Gynaecologic Oncologic Surgical Procedures Manual para-aortic dissection consists of resection of the nodal tissue over the distal vena cava from the level of inferior mesenteric artery (IMA) to the mid-right common iliac artery and between aorta and left ureter from the IMA to left mid common iliac artery. However, all the lymphatics follow the vessels and on the right side the ovarian vessels open into the IVC and into the renal vein on the left. So the lymphatics follow the same and in case of high-risk cases for para-aortic nodal involvement, it is the nodes between the renal vein and IMA which is important and not the ones below the IMA. Studies have shown approximately 77% of patients with para-aortic nodal involvement are found to have metastases above the level of the IMA, and 63% of patients with positive nodes below the IMA also have positive nodes above the IMA (**Fig. 10.5**).[10,43] Metastatic spread to the upper para-aortic nodes between the IMA and renal vessels without involvement of the lower para-aortic nodes or common iliac nodes has been described.[10] Thus,

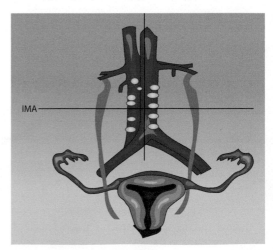

Fig. 10.5   Metastasis above inferior mesenteric artery (IMA) 77%.

limiting dissection of para-aortic nodes to the level of the IMA may potentially miss 38 to 46% of patients with positive para-aortic nodes. In order to identify nodes present at distant sites, particularly above the IMA, systematic pelvic and para-aortic lymphadenectomy, with dissection optimally carried out to the renal vessels, is important in high-risk patients.[10]

Pomel's Classification System for Para-aortic Node Dissection[44]

A. **Systematic para-aortic node dissection**
  A1. Complete (includes infrarenal and suprarenal up to the coeliac trunk to midpoint of common iliac vessels).
  A2. Infrarenal (as above, but does not include suprarenal dissection).
  A3. Infra-IMA (as above, but does not include dissection above IMA).
B. **Para-aortic node sampling**
  B1. Extensive.
  B2. Minimal.
C. **Nonexcisional assessment**
  C1. Palpation (direct), following full exposure of para-aortic areas.
  C2. Palpation (indirect), transperitoneal without any exposure.
  C3. Radiological assessment by (PET)/ computed tomography (CT), CT or magnetic resonance imaging (MRI).

Technique

Retroperitoneal LND can be by open, laparoscopic, and robotic techniques.

For pelvic lymphadenectomy all three approaches are easy. Laparoscopic para-aortic lymphadenectomy can be done by transperitoneal and extraperitoneal approach but is difficult to master due to rigid instruments, lack of endowrist, and falling mesentery. In patients with high BMI, open technique has increased morbidity.

Hence, the development of robotic technique has the advantages of stereotopic vision, 12× magnification, endowrist, excellent vision, multitasking instrument, availability of four instruments, and easy suturing from both right and left hands.

Preoperative Preparation

Patient takes diet up to 8 hours prior to surgery. Deep vein thrombosis (DVT) prophylaxis is given on the night before. Carboload is given orally 2 hours before surgery as a part of ERAS protocol. The author does not practice mechanical bowel preparation.

Position of the Patient

Extreme Trendelenburg: Keeping the right leg up allows space for the third arm.

Port Placement and Instrumentation

Vaginal–Cervical Ahluwalia Retractor-Elevator (V-CARE) uterine manipulator (ConMed endosurgery, Utica, NY) is used to manipulate the uterus intraoperatively but is not mandatory.

A 12mm camera port is placed 3 cm above the umbilicus in the midline with optical trocar. Arm one (8 mm) port is placed on patient's right side, 3 to 5 cm below and at least 8 cm lateral to camera port. Arm two (8 mm) port is placed on patient's left side, 8 cm lateral and 3 to 5 cm below the level of the camera port.

Third arm (8 mm) is placed on patient's left side, 2 cm above anterior superior iliac spine, and 8 cm away from the second port. Assistant port (12 mm) is placed on patient's right side, slightly cephalad to the camera port on an arc at the midpoint between the camera port and the instrument arm one port. Zero-degree scope is used for all the steps, except for para-aortic LND where 30 degrees down scope is used. In arm one hot shears (monopolar curved scissors), in arm two fenestrated bipolar forceps, and in arm three prograsp forceps are used.

Surgical Steps of Robotic Pelvic Lymphadenectomy (Fig. 10.6)

The authors choose to use hot shears with curved scissors connected to monopolar in the right hand and Maryland or fenestrated grasper with bipolar in the left hand.

The steps of the procedure include:
- The peritoneum is incised along the psoas muscle lateral to the level of the pelvic vessels and retroperitoneum is accessed. Any adhesion if present especially on the left side is divided sharply.

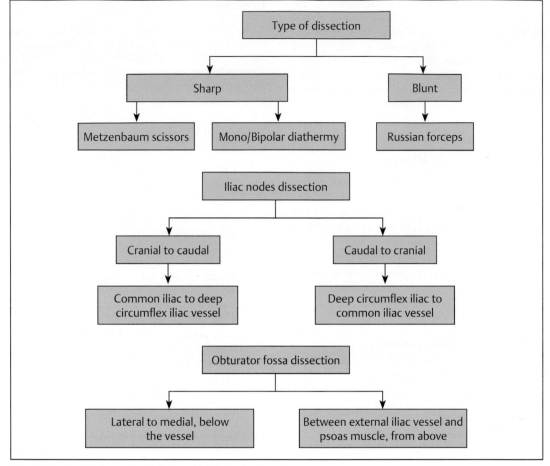

Fig. 10.6   Surgical steps of robotic pelvic lymphadenectomy.

- The round ligaments are transected. This allows better exposure of the obturator fossa and the distal external iliac vessels.
- The pararectal and paravesical spaces are then developed.

Paravesical space is defined as the space between obliterated umbilical artery medially and external iliac vessels laterally. The obliterated umbilical artery is usually visualized as a discrete fold on either side of the bladder. Developing the area between the obliterated umbilical artery and the external iliac vessels exposes the paravesical space medially and the obturator fossa laterally. Cut the peritoneal reflection above till the common iliac artery.

- The ureter is identified along the medial peritoneal fold. This is typically retracted medially during the entire procedure.

- The pararectal space can be developed between the ureter medially and the internal iliac artery laterally.
- Dissection can be cranial to caudal or vice versa.
- The pelvic LND is then initiated by dissecting the lateral nodal tissue away from the psoas muscle. Care is taken to identify and isolate the genitofemoral nerve, which can easily be mistaken to be a lymphatic channel.
- The dissection continues until the circumflex iliac vein inferiorly, which is the distal-most boundary of the pelvic node dissection. Deep circumflex iliac vein, which lies below the inguinal ligament, is a tributary which crosses the external iliac

artery and drains into the external iliac vein medially.

- At this point, the sheath of the external iliac artery is incised, and the fibrofatty tissue surrounding the external iliac vessels is elevated.
- The tissue is then swung lateral to the medial.
- The surgeon then dissects within the obturator fossa. The pelvic side wall formed by the obturator internus is exposed. Attention should be given to the iliolumbar trunk of nerves from the sacral plexus.
- The fibrofatty tissue of the lymph node bundle is retracted medially, and a plane is created underneath the external iliac vein. Sharp and blunt dissection is performed within the fossa until the obturator nerve is visualized; this nerve can be isolated along its entire course within the obturator fossa. It is prudent to use minimal cautery at this juncture.
- In 15 to 20 percent of patients, accessory vessels may arise in this space from the undersurface of the external iliac vein. These must be clipped or cauterized only after the obturator nerve is identified and well delineated with the ureter safely retracted out of the field of dissection.
- Extending the dissection cranially the fork of the common iliac vessels is defined, and all the fibrofatty tissues at this site are removed.
- The entire fibrofatty tissue with all the lymphatics and lymph nodes should be excised in toto in endobag.
- Similar procedure is repeated on the opposite side.
- There is no change of instruments in the entire surgery with a binocular 3D view and 10× magnification, endowrist.

Surgical Steps of Para-aortic Lymphadenectomy (Fig. 10.7)

In high-risk EC after radical hysterectomy and systematic pelvic lymphadenectomy, high para-aortic nodal dissection up to renal veins is required.

- If central docking is done, the arms don't reach high para-aortic region up to renal veins.
- If side docking is done, it is not optimal for pelvic surgery.
- Most of the times dual docking or change of position of both patient and robot is required.
- Intuitive recommended procedure card and port placement is suboptimal in achieving this.

Hence, the author (Somashekhar SP and team) has devised his own modified innovative ports

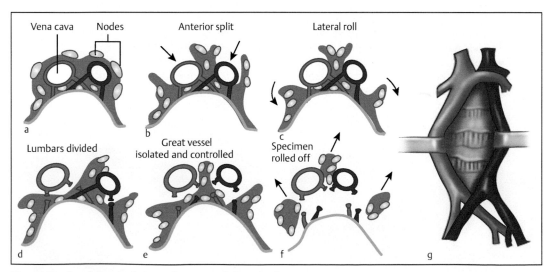

Fig. 10.7   (a–g) Surgical steps of para-aortic lymphadenectomy.

placement technique which is ideal for both pelvic and para-aortic lymphadenectomy.

Modified Innovative Port Placement

- Very high camera port in epigastrium.
- Two ports on the right side, so two graspers.

Modified Centroside Docking

- Area is available for V-care intrauterine manipulation.
- Both arms can reach left renal veins.
- Single docking and same pelvic ports.
- Neither patient nor robot changes the position.

In robotic surgery, reaching the pelvis from the epigastrium is not a problem as instruments are long but staying too close to the target organ is always a mistake (**Figs. 10.8** and **10.9**).

Midline split and lateral roll technique is followed. A 30-degree down camera is used. The right hand (R1) has hot shears and the left hand fenestrated bipolar (R2). Hook is also a helpful instrument while doing para-aortic dissection.

- Step 1: On the aorta and IVC, midline split is done, which takes care of preaortic, precaval, and some portion of interaortocaval lymph nodes. Between the IMA and aorta, the hypogastric plexus is preserved carefully.
- Step 2: Now we do the lateral roll technique.

The camera is changed to a 0-degree camera and turned one-fourth anticlockwise. Hot shears are changed to left hand, R2. This prevents the hood from obstructing the view and enables us to view behind the IVC and aorta. Fenestrated bipolars are now in right hand, R1. The aorta and IVC are visualized from lateral area. The psoas muscle is defined on the right side and the ovarian pedicles dip into the IVC below the renal vessels. Anatomy until the renal vein is defined. All the structures are visualized parallel. The paracaval, retrocaval, retroaortic, and interaortocaval nodal packet are dissected out. It is essential to identify and preserve the fellow's vein; one is two inches above the division of the common iliac vein and one on the right paracaval. It is advisable to go between the interaortocaval area until the glistening anterior spinal ligament is demonstrated. All the aspects of aortic groups—the right paracaval, left paracaval, preaortic, para-aortic, retrocaval, and retroaortic—can be taken.

The whole surgery can be done without a change in the position of the robot or instruments.

Analysis of Demographic and Unpaired Data

- See **Table 10.1**.[39]

Sentinel Lymph Node Biopsy

An SLN is defined as a lymph node directly connected to the primary tumor through a lymphatic channel. It is the lymph node(s) most likely first to receive metastases from the primary tumor.

SLN is becoming much more accepted in treatment of endometrial and cervical cancer and has been addressed in guidelines from the Society of Gynecologic Oncology.[45]

The rationale for SLN mapping is to:

- Classify patients with lymph node metastases and avoid the morbidity of a complete lymphadenectomy.
- SLN mapping may also be considered a technique that may identify occult metastatic disease if the node lies outside of the usual boundaries of pelvic or para-aortic LND.

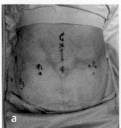
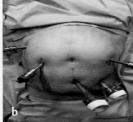

Fig. 10.8   (a, b) Port placement.

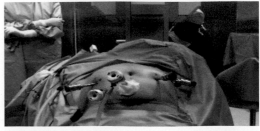

Fig. 10.9   Para-aortic lymph node dissection.

Table 10.1   Analysis of demographic and unpaired data

Variable	Robotic surgery	Open surgery	p-value
Age, y	61.44	62.80	0.535
Operating time, min	119.2	180.2	<0.001
Estimated blood loss, mL	81.28	234	<0.001
Number of lymph nodes removed	17.5	11.6	0.071
Hospital stay, d	1.94	5.54	<0.001
Postoperative complications (minor)	0	5	0.050
Postoperative complications (major)	0	0	1.00

- Also, the SLN evaluation process typically includes ultrasection of the SLN and immunohistochemical staining, which may be more sensitive than the traditional hematoxylin and eosin evaluation.

SLNB has become a standard for the management of the retroperitoneal lymph nodes in EC.

The FIRES trial was a multicenter, prospective cohort study comparing SLNB to lymphadenectomy for EC staging. It showed sensitivity of 97.2% with negative predictive value of 99.6%. It concluded that SLN by Indocyanine green (ICG) can safely replace lymphadenectomy in EC.[46,47] The NCCN up-to-date endometrial staging[48] and the SGO[49] also back the role of sentinel lymphadenectomy in EC.

In cervical cancer, role of SLN is promising but still investigational.[50,51] In a French study, the procedure was found to have a sensitivity of 92% and negative predictive value of 98%.[52]

- Technique of SLN dissection: At Manipal hospital ICG diluted to 1.25 mg/mL concentration is injected 1 mL into the superficial (2 mm) and deep (1 cm) cervical stroma at 3 and 9 o'clock positions each. After docking, the nodes are visualized in firefly mode. Successful mapping of a hemipelvis is defined by observing a channel leading from the cervix directly to at least one candidate lymph node. Common iliac or aortic SLNs are also dissected if present. Identified SLNs are then retrieved and sent for pathologic evaluation.
- In a study by Somashekhar et al, the overall detection rate of ICG-based SLN was

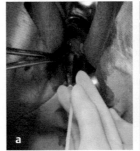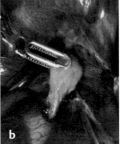

Fig. 10.10   **(a)** ICG dye being injected. **(b)** ICG dye directed SLN.

98% in a cohort of 100 cases of carcinoma endometrium which underwent robotic-assisted Type 1 pan-hysterectomy, with ICG-directed sentinel lymph node (SLN) biopsy.[53]

Utilizing a standardized strategy when intending to perform an SLND in patients with EC has been shown to improve the SLND detection rate and decrease the rate of complete pelvic LND (**Figs. 10.10** and **10.11**).[47,49]

Tips and Tricks for Safe Robotic Pelvic and Para-aortic Nodal Dissection

- Position: Trendelenburg.
- Coordination and sync with the anesthetist: The hydration should be kept low

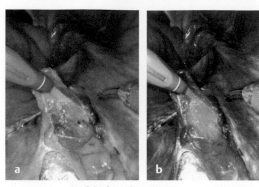

Fig. 10.11 **(a, b)** Identifying SLN.

so that the veins are collapsed. The anesthetist is requested to keep the central venous pressure (CVP) low so that the IVC is not distended. It is essential to understand that arterial bleed is high pressure and low volume and can be tackled with bipolar easily. The venous ooze is a greater enemy as it is low pressure and high volume. This can lead to hemodynamic instability, and every attempt should be made to avoid this. Lest this happens, it should be clipped or sutured; veins don't take bipolar due to thinner tunica media.

- Exposure: Good exposure is the key. The mesentery can be retracted using T-lift, versa band, or rubber retraction technique.
- Identification and knowing the levels of fellow's vein: It is crucial to identify and ligate the two fellow's vein to avoid bleeding. The first fellow's vein is one inch above the common iliac vein confluence and the second one lies one inch above the first one draining into the anterior surface of IVC.
- Identifying the lumbar vein: Beware of the lumbar veins while doing paracaval and retrocaval lymphadenectomy because they have no valves and bleed from both ends. Suture ligation is the only way to control this bleed.
- Identifying abnormal anatomy of the renal artery: This can help prevent avoidable bleeding.
- It is imperative to identify and preserve the artery of Adamkiewicz over the anterior spinal ligament. Lack of flow to this vessel can cause ischemia to the spinal cord.

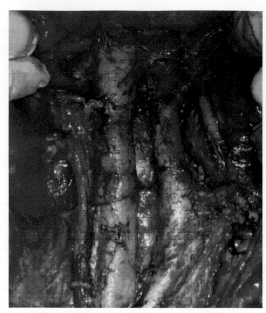

Fig. 10.12 Fork node lying between left renal vein and aorta.

- Before the start of the procedure it is advisable to park a rolled gauze intra-abdominally. In case of bleeding, gauze is used to give compression with the third arm while waiting for a minimum of two clotting times (2 × 3.5 s). As the anesthetist stabilizes the patient, needle drive can be taken for suture ligation.
- It is essential to know that the paracaval and retrocaval nodes are the most common nodes involved.
- The fork node which lies between the left renal vein and border of aorta is very commonly involved and should not be left behind (**Fig. 10.12**).

Complications

- Major vascular injury.
- Symptomatic lymphocele.
- Chylous ascites.
- Paralytic ileus/delayed bowel recovery.
- Ureteric injury.
- Fistulas.
- Blood transfusions.
- Bowel injuries.
- Lower limb lymphedema.

Management of Bleeding and Vascular Injuries

- Keep the blood pressure and CVP low.
- For any bleeding, wait for two clotting times.
- Keep a preloaded suture ready (preferably 4–0 Prolene with two knots at the end which snuggly fits and seals the rent in the IVC).
- Do not use monopolar or bipolar cautery, it may increase the rent. It is preferable to use a suture or clip (not hemolock) (**Fig. 10.13**).

Management of Chylous Ascites

Chylous ascites are not same as chyle leak. It results from injury to major cisterna chyli and lumbar lymphatics. If not treated, chylous ascites has a high mortality.

The cisterna chyli is formed by the junction of the left and right lumbar, intestinal, and descending intercostal lumbar trunks at L1 and L2 vertebral levels immediately to the right of the aorta behind the right crus of the diaphragm.

- Ligating all the lymphatics carefully.
- The leak can be low volume or high volume, which should be quantified.
- Diet modification with medium-chain triglycerides should be tried for 1 week.
- If the leak still does not subside, use ICG in the first web space of the foot or lymphangiogram to locate the lymphatic leak.
- Once the leak is localized, it can be sealed using a lipoidal or coil by the interventional radiologist.

If this fails, a robotic or laparoscopic procedure can be done to suture ligate or clip the leak. During the procedure, the patient is given a fatty meal through the Ryles tube with or without ICG to locate the leaking duct which can then be easily ligated.

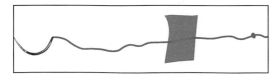

Fig. 10.13 4–0 Prolene with surgical and knot in the end.

Learning Curve

The learning curve is usually defined as the number of cases that a surgeon needs to perform before reaching competency for a given procedure based on comparisons with the outcomes of prior standard procedures.[54] The earlier studies have used the following end points in assessing the learning curve in open and laparoscopic surgeries:

- Estimated blood loss.
- Conversion rate.
- Duration of hospitalization.

Later on, as a measure of the learning curve, studies have focused on:

- Docking time.
- Console time.
- OR time.
- Lymph nodes harvest.

In the study by Somashekhar et al,[55] an adequate number of pelvic lymph nodes retrieval of 12 was achieved by the ninth case, and consistently, more number of pelvic nodes were removed, and para-aortic lymph nodes retrieval of 10 was achieved after the eighteenth case.

Ways to shorten the learning curve:

- Structured robotic training program.
- Proctoring and mentoring.
- To figure out the optimal patient positioning.
- To figure out the optimal angle of robot docking.
- To figure out the optimal port placements.
- To figure out the optimal tissue handling.
- To break down the surgery into a series of steps and master each step (parallel learning).
- Self-auditing of the surgeries done.
- Peer/online review of the surgeries performed.
- Dual console.
- Proper patient selection.
- Trial discussion and planning of surgery by the team a day before.
- Discussion of the steps of surgery and reviewing the critical steps, including the video discussion.
- Support staff and other involved faculties (anesthesiologists, nursing staff) made aware of the surgery a day prior.
- Standardizing the port placement techniques.

- Protocols to be fixed regarding the steps of surgery.
- Frequent use of simulators by surgeons and regular practice.
- Proper communication between the console surgeon and the bedside assistant.

The CUSUM chart is for surgeon console time (**Fig. 10.14**). CUSUM chart analysis is an effective and powerful statistical tool for determining if and when a change in a data set has occurred. The direction of CUSUM line changes at 12th case, which is the indication that surgeon docking time has started reducing; thus, it is the cutoff point of a learning curve. Further the CUSUM line maintains the downward trend signifies surgeon console time consistently kept lower than the target time.

Advantages of Robotic Surgery

- Shorter learning curve than laparoscopic surgery.
- Not counterintuitive.
- Vision is magnified and is 3D increased depth perception: Stereoscopic.
- Eliminates assistant-held laparoscope and resultant tremor: Stability.
- Endowristed instrumentation: Superior precision (allows for easier sewing and

more complex dissections—reduced conversion rate).
- Nondominant hand surgery.
- Fewer complications, blood loss, blood transfusions than laparoscopic surgery.
- Motion-dampening sensors prevent torqueing at port sites and therefore less patient discomfort.
- Stable surgeon-controlled instruments: tremor reduction.
- Ergonomic: Less fatigue.

Conclusion

- Lymphadenectomy is an integral part of gynecology oncology procedures.
- Pelvic lymphadenectomy alone is not sufficient for high-risk endometrial and ovarian cancer as the most common site of lymphatic spread is above the IMA up to renal vein by venous drainage.
- Para-aortic lymphadenectomy is technically demanding in laparoscopy. In comparison, robotic retroperitoneal lymph node dissection is easy with a short learning curve, less conversion rate, single docking, easy reproducibility, and excellent lymph nodal yield.

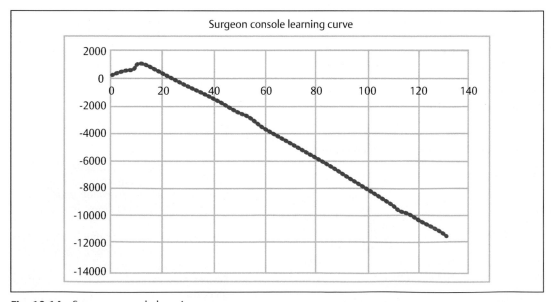

Fig. 10.14   Surgeon console learning curve.

- Robotic-assisted surgery and open surgery for systematic high para-aortic lymphadenectomy has the same oncological outcomes, as far as the completeness of systematic surgical staging is concerned.
- But in addition to this, robotic procedure has all the advantages of minimal invasive technique and benefits to patient.
- Our unique technique of port placement and single docking technique enables both pelvic and high robotic para-aortic lymphadenectomy easy.
- LND is not inferior to the open method.
- Blood loss, hospital stay, and pain were less.
- Quicker recovery and early return to normal activities.
- Smaller incision and improved cosmesis.
- Better clinical outcome and patient satisfaction.

References

1. Somashekhar SP. Does debulking of enlarged positive lymph nodes improve survival in different gynaecological cancers? Best Pract Res Clin Obstet Gynaecol 2015;29(6):870–883
2. Creasman WT, Morrow CP, Bundy BN, Homesley HD, Graham JE, Heller PB. Surgical pathologic spread patterns of endometrial cancer. A Gynecologic Oncology Group Study. Cancer 1987; 60(8, Suppl):2035–2041
3. Benedetti Panici P, Basile S, Maneschi F, et al. Systematic pelvic lymphadenectomy vs. no lymphadenectomy in early-stage endometrial carcinoma: randomized clinical trial. J Natl Cancer Inst 2008;100(23):1707–1716
4. Kitchener H, Swart AM, Qian Q, Amos C, Parmar MK; ASTEC study group. Efficacy of systematic pelvic lymphadenectomy in endometrial cancer (MRC ASTEC trial): a randomised study. Lancet 2009;373(9658):125–136
5. Todo Y, Kato H, Kaneuchi M, Watari H, Takeda M, Sakuragi N. Survival effect of para-aortic lymphadenectomy in endometrial cancer (SEPAL study): a retrospective cohort analysis. Lancet 2010;375(9721):1165–1172
6. Todo Y, Yamamoto R, Minobe S, et al. Risk factors for postoperative lower-extremity lymphedema in endometrial cancer survivors who had treatment including lymphadenectomy. Gynecol Oncol 2010;119(1):60–64

7. Abu-Rustum NR, Alektiar K, Iasonos A, et al. The incidence of symptomatic lower-extremity lymphedema following treatment of uterine corpus malignancies: a 12-year experience at Memorial Sloan-Kettering Cancer Center. Gynecol Oncol 2006;103(2):714–718
8. Kumar S, Podratz KC, Bakkum-Gamez JN, et al. Prospective assessment of the prevalence of pelvic, paraaortic and high paraaortic lymph node metastasis in endometrial cancer. Gynecol Oncol 2014;132(1):38–43
9. Talukdar S, Kumar S, Bhatla N, Mathur S, Thulkar S, Kumar L. Neo-adjuvant chemotherapy in the treatment of advanced malignant germ cell tumors of ovary. Gynecol Oncol 2014; 132(1):28–32
10. Mariani A, Dowdy SC, Cliby WA, et al. Prospective assessment of lymphatic dissemination in endometrial cancer: a paradigm shift in surgical staging. Gynecol Oncol 2008;109(1):11–18 10.1016/j.ygyno.2008.01.023
11. Mariani A, Webb MJ, Keeney GL, Haddock MG, Calori G, Podratz KC. Low-risk corpus cancer: is lymphadenectomy or radiotherapy necessary? Am J Obstet Gynecol 2000;182(6):1506–1519
12. Vargas R, Rauh-Hain JA, Clemmer J, et al. Tumor size, depth of invasion, and histologic grade as prognostic factors of lymph node involvement in endometrial cancer: a SEER analysis. Gynecol Oncol 2014;133(2):216–220
13. AlHilli MM, Mariani A. Preoperative selection of endometrial cancer patients at low risk for lymph node metastases: useful criteria for enrollment in clinical trials. J Gynecol Oncol 2014;25(4):267–269
14. Kumar S, Mariani A, Bakkum-Gamez JN, et al. Risk factors that mitigate the role of paraaortic lymphadenectomy in uterine endometrioid cancer. Gynecol Oncol 2013;130(3):441–445
15. Gold MA, Tian C, Whitney CW, Rose PG, Lanciano R. Surgical versus radiographic determination of para-aortic lymph node metastases before chemoradiation for locally advanced cervical carcinoma: a Gynecologic Oncology Group Study. Cancer 2008;112(9):1954–1963
16. Reynolds EA, Tierney K, Keeney GL, et al. Analysis of outcomes of microinvasive adenocarcinoma of the uterine cervix by treatment type. Obstet Gynecol 2010;116(5):1150–1157
17. Committee on Practice Bulletins-Gynecology. ACOG practice bulletin. Diagnosis and treatment of cervical carcinomas, number 35, May 2002. Obstet Gynecol 2002;99(5 Pt 1):855–867
18. Benedet JL, Anderson GH. Stage IA carcinoma of the cervix revisited. Obstet Gynecol 1996; 87(6):1052–1059

19. Hughes RR, Brewington KC, Hanjani P, et al. Extended field irradiation for cervical cancer based on surgical staging. Gynecol Oncol 1980;9(2):153–161

20. Greer BE, Koh WJ, Abu-Rustum NR, et al; National Comprehensive Cancer Networks. Cervical cancer. J Natl Compr Canc Netw 2010; 8(12):1388–1416

21. Rose PG, Bundy BN, Watkins EB, et al. Concurrent cisplatin-based radiotherapy and chemotherapy for locally advanced cervical cancer. N Engl J Med 1999;340(15):1144–1153

22. Peters WA III, Liu PY, Barrett RJ II, et al. Concurrent chemotherapy and pelvic radiation therapy compared with pelvic radiation therapy alone as adjuvant therapy after radical surgery in high-risk early-stage cancer of the cervix. J Clin Oncol 2000;18(8):1606–1613

23. Moore KN, Gold MA, McMeekin DS, Walker JL, Rutledge T, Zorn KK. Extraperitoneal para-aortic lymph node evaluation for cervical cancer via pfannenstiel incision: technique and peri-operative outcomes. Gynecol Oncol 2008;108(3):466–471

24. Weiser EB, Bundy BN, Hoskins WJ, et al. Extraperitoneal versus transperitoneal selective paraaortic lymphadenectomy in the pretreatment surgical staging of advanced cervical carcinoma (a Gynecologic Oncology Group study). Gynecol Oncol 1989;33(3): 283–289

25. Abu-Rustum NR, Yashar CM, Bean S, et al. NCCN Guidelines Insights: Cervical Cancer, Version 1. 2020. J Natl Compr Canc Netw 2020; 18(6):660–666

26. Krasner C, Duska L. Management of women with newly diagnosed ovarian cancer. Semin Oncol 2009;36(2):91–105

27. Koulouris CR, Penson RT. Ovarian stromal and germ cell tumors. Semin Oncol 2009;36(2): 126–136

28. Burghardt E, Girardi F, Lahousen M, Tamussino K, Stettner H. Patterns of pelvic and paraaortic lymph node involvement in ovarian cancer. Gynecol Oncol 1991;40(2):103–106

29. Berek JS. Lymph node-positive stage IIIC ovarian cancer: a separate entity? Int J Gynecol Cancer 2009;19(Suppl 2):S18–S20

30. Aletti GD, Dowdy S, Podratz KC, Cliby WA. Role of lymphadenectomy in the management of grossly apparent advanced stage epithelial ovarian cancer. Am J Obstet Gynecol 2006; 195(6):1862–1868

31. du Bois A, Reuss A, Harter P, Pujade-Lauraine E, Ray-Coquard I, Pfisterer J; Arbeitsgemeinschaft Gynaekologische Onkologie Studiengruppe Ovarialkarzinom; Groupe d'Investigateurs Nationaux pour l'Etude des Cancers Ovariens. Potential role of lymphadenectomy in advanced ovarian cancer: a combined exploratory analysis of three prospectively randomized phase III multicenter trials. J Clin Oncol 2010;28(10):1733–1739

32. Panici PB, Maggioni A, Hacker N, et al. Systematic aortic and pelvic lymphadenectomy versus resection of bulky nodes only in optimally debulked advanced ovarian cancer: a randomized clinical trial. J Natl Cancer Inst 2005;97(8):560–566

33. Harter P, Sehouli J, Lorusso D, et al. A Randomized Trial of Lymphadenectomy in Patients with Advanced Ovarian Neoplasms. N Engl J Med 2019;380(9):822–832

34. Walker JL, Piedmonte MR, Spirtos NM, et al. Laparoscopy compared with laparotomy for comprehensive surgical staging of uterine cancer: Gynecologic Oncology Group Study LAP2. J Clin Oncol 2009;27(32):5331–5336

35. Janda M, Gebski V, Davies LC, et al. Effect of Total Laparoscopic Hysterectomy vs Total Abdominal Hysterectomy on Disease-Free Survival Among Women With Stage I Endometrial Cancer: A Randomized Clinical Trial. JAMA 2017;317(12):1224–1233

36. Cusimano MC, Simpson AN, Dossa F, et al. Laparoscopic and robotic hysterectomy in endometrial cancer patients with obesity: a systematic review and meta-analysis of conversions and complications. Am J Obstet Gynecol 2019;221(5):410–428.e19

37. Mäenpää MM, Nieminen K, Tomás EI, Laurila M, Luukkaala TH, Mäenpää JU. Robotic-assisted vs traditional laparoscopic surgery for endometrial cancer: a randomized controlled trial. Am J Obstet Gynecol 2016;215(5):588. e1–588.e7

38. Wright JD, Burke WM, Wilde ET, et al. Comparative effectiveness of robotic versus laparoscopic hysterectomy for endometrial cancer. J Clin Oncol 2012;30(8):783–791

39. Somashekhar SP, Jaka RC, Zaveri SS. Prospective randomized study comparing robotic-assisted hysterectomy and regional lymphadenectomy with traditional laparotomy for staging of endometrial carcinoma—initial Indian experience. Indian J Surg Oncol 2014;5(3):217–223

40. Lécuru F, Neji K, Robin F, Darles C, de Bièvre P, Taurelle R. Lymphatic drainage of the uterus. Preliminary results of an experimental study. J Gynecol Obstet Biol Reprod (Paris) 1997;26(4):418–423

41. Whitney CW, Spirtos N. Gynecologic Oncology Group surgical procedures manual. Philadelphia: Gynecologic Oncology Group; 2010

42. Ben Shachar I, Fowler JM. The role of laparoscopy in the management of gynecologic cancers. In: Gershenson DM, Gore M, McGuire WP, et al., eds. Gynecologic Cancer: Controversies in Mangement. London: Churchill Livingstone; 2004

43. Mariani A, Dowdy SC, Cliby WA, et al. Prospective assessment of lymphatic dissemination in endometrial cancer: a paradigm shift in surgical staging. Gynecol Oncol 2008;109(1):11–18

44. Pomel C, Naik R, Martinez A, et al. Systematic (complete) para-aortic lymphadenectomy: description of a novel surgical classification with technical and anatomical considerations. BJOG 2012;119(2):249–253

45. Ramirez PT, Jhingran A, Macapinlac HA, et al. Laparoscopic extraperitoneal para-aortic lymphadenectomy in locally advanced cervical cancer: a prospective correlation of surgical findings with positron emission tomography/ computed tomography findings. Cancer 2011; 117(9):1928–1934

46. Rossi EC, Kowalski LD, Scalici J, et al. A comparison of sentinel lymph node biopsy to lymphadenectomy for endometrial cancer staging (FIRES trial): a multicentre, prospective, cohort study. Lancet Oncol 2017;18(3):384–392

47. Ballester M, Dubernard G, Lécuru F, et al. Detection rate and diagnostic accuracy of sentinel-node biopsy in early stage endometrial cancer: a prospective multicentre study (SENTI-ENDO). Lancet Oncol 2011;12(5):469–476

48. NCCN Clinical Practice Guidelines in Oncology. Uterine Neoplasms. http://www.nccn.org/ professionals/physician_gls/pdf/uterine.pdf

49. Holloway RW, Abu-Rustum NR, Backes FJ, et al. Sentinel lymph node mapping and staging in endometrial cancer: a Society of Gynecologic Oncology literature review with consensus recommendations. Gynecol Oncol 2017;146(2):405–415

50. Frumovitz M, Ramirez PT, Levenback CF. Lymphatic mapping and sentinel lymph node detection in women with cervical cancer. Gynecol Oncol 2008; 110(3, Suppl 2):S17–S20

51. Kim CH, Soslow RA, Park KJ, et al. Pathologic ultrastaging improves micrometastasis detection in sentinel lymph nodes during endometrial cancer staging. Int J Gynecol Cancer 2013;23(5):964–970

52. Barlin JN, Khoury-Collado F, Kim CH, et al. The importance of applying a sentinel lymph node mapping algorithm in endometrial cancer staging: beyond removal of blue nodes. Gynecol Oncol 2012;125(3):531–535

53. Somashekhar SP, Arvind R, Kumar CR, Ahuja V, Ashwin KR. Sentinel node mapping using indocyanine green and near-infrared fluorescence imaging technology for endometrial cancer: a prospective study using a surgical algorithm in Indian patients. J Min Access Surg [Epub ahead of print] [cited 2021 Jun 21]. Available from: https://www.journalofmas.com/preprintarticle.asp?id=309085

54. Park IJ, Choi GS, Lim KH, Kang BM, Jun SH. Multidimensional analysis of the learning curve for laparoscopic colorectal surgery: lessons from 1,000 cases of laparoscopic colorectal surgery. Surg Endosc 2009;23(4):839–846

55. Jacob SS, Somashekhar SP, Jaka R, Ashwin KR, Kumar R. Robotic-assisted pelvic and high para-aortic lymphadenectomy (RPLND) for endometrial cancer and learning curve. Indian Journal of Gynecologic Oncology 2016;14(2)

Accompanying Videos

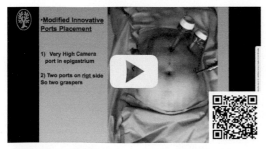

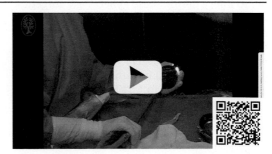

Video 10.1 Robotic para-aortic lymphadenectomy. https://www.thieme.de/de/q.htm?p=opn/cs/21/6/15245410-7c9da0d5

Video 10.2 Robotic PLND. https://www.thieme.de/de/q.htm?p=opn/cs/21/6/15245531-63eaaca2

11 Identifying and Preventing Ureteric Injuries in Complex Gynecologic Surgeries

Sunil Kumar and Shiv Charan Navriya

Abstract

Ureter traverses through retroperitoneum in the abdomen and extraperitoneal space of pelvic cavity. It has a close relationship with pelvic organs. Hence, the ureter is susceptible to injury during gynecologic surgeries like hysterectomy, myomectomy, endometriectomy, and surgery for pelvic tumors. A sound knowledge of location and identification of ureter during gynecologic surgery is of paramount importance as missed ureteric injury can have serious consequences on the function of renal unit and may result in significant rate of morbidity in such patients.

Introduction

Hysterectomy, myomectomy, ovarian tumor excision, endometriectomy, and salpingectomy are commonly performed surgeries in gynecology. Because of proximity of ureter to internal genital organs in the pelvic cavity, it is susceptible to injury during these gynecologic surgeries. Whereas the incidence of ureteric injury during open and laparoscopic gynecologic surgery is 0.5 to 2.5%, a true incidence of ureteric injury during robotic gynecologic surgery is unknown. The incidence of ureteric trauma during gynecologic surgery ranges from 0.1 to 1.5% for benign cases and ≤5% for oncological procedures. Hysterectomy is the most common cause of ureteric injury.[1,2] Ureteric injuries during robotic gynecologic surgery are assumed to be well below than in laparoscopic surgery because of several reasons such as robotic surgery is done in a 3D vision,

ergonomics is better, surgeon fatigue is less, there is the absence of tremor and better control over the movement of instruments because of scaling of motion, and there is seven degrees of freedom of movement which makes precise and fine dissection of tissue plane possible.

Relevant Anatomy of the Ureter

The adult ureter is 22 to 30 cm in length and spans from the kidney to urinary bladder in the retroperitoneal space of abdomen and the extraperitoneal space of the pelvic cavity. As seen laparoscopically, the ureter can be divided into abdominal (from the renal pelvis to iliac vessel) and pelvic (from iliac vessel to bladder) segments. The pelvic part of the ureter constitutes almost half (15 cm) of its total length. The intramural segment of ureter is 1.2 to 2.5 cm in length. In retroperitoneal space, ureter lies over the psoas muscle and runs parallel and posterior to the ovarian vessel (**Fig. 11.1**).

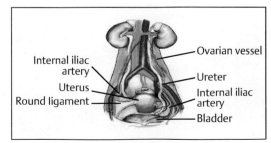

Fig. 11.1 Course and relation of ureter in retroperitoneum and pelvis.

Near pelvic brim, ovarian vessels cross anterior to the ureter contained in the suspensory ligament of the ovary. Ureter travels anterior to the bifurcation of iliac artery near the pelvic brim to enter the true pelvic cavity and courses laterally along the pelvic wall. Here it lies in close relation to uterosacral ligament and passes posterior to the ovary to form the posterior boundary of the ovarian fossa. At the level of internal os, ureter lies 2 cm lateral to supravaginal portion of cervix beneath the uterine artery in the parametrial connective tissue (cardinal ligament; **Figs. 11.2** and **11.3**). This is the most vulnerable location of injury to ureter during hysterectomy. The terminal ureter runs forward, accompanied by the neurovascular bundle of the bladder and passes the anterior vaginal fornix just before entering the bladder. This proximity of the ureter to the uterine vessels is the cause of ureteral injuries during hysterectomy.[3–9]

Ureter receives multiple small arterial branches from renal artery, abdominal aorta, gonadal artery, iliac artery, and superior and inferior vesical artery (**Fig. 11.1**). These arteries anastomose extensively in periureteral adventitial tissue. Venous drainage occurs through multiple tributaries into renal, gonadal, and internal iliac veins. It is important to preserve this periureteral adventitial tissue while mobilizing the ureter. Striping off this adventitial tissue results in ischemia and subsequent stricture of ureter.[10,11]

Susceptible Points of Ureteric Injury

Following are critical sites of possible ureteral injury during gynecologic surgery:

- Infundibulopelvic (IP) ligament.

- Lateral border of the uterosacral ligament.
- Cardinal ligament.
- Along its course near the anterior vaginal wall.

Cardinal ligament is the most common site of ureteric injury during gynecologic surgery. However, during laparoscopic surgery, ureter is most susceptible to injury at IP ligament, in the ovarian fossa, and in the ureteric canal.[12,13]

Risk Factors for Ureteral Injury

The incidence of ureteral injury in radical hysterectomy for malignant conditions like uterine and ovarian cancer is higher than in hysterectomy for benign diseases like endometriosis, dysfunctional uterine bleeding, leiomyoma, and prolapse.[14] Pelvic inflammatory disease, previous pelvic surgery, history of pelvic radiation, and congenital anomalies are risk factors for ureteral injury during hysterectomy.[15] However, there is no identifiable cause in about 50% of cases of ureteral injury during hysterectomy. Intraoperative bleeding is an important cause of ureteral injury where the surgeon may inadvertently ligate or cause thermal injury in an attempt to control bleeding.

Risk Factors of Ureteral Injury during Hysterectomy

- Malignant conditions like uterine and ovarian cancers.
- Endometriosis.
- Pelvic inflammatory disease.
- History of pelvic radiation.
- Congenital anomalies.
- Uncontrolled bleeding.

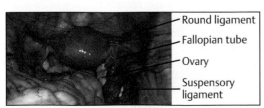

Fig. 11.2 Panoramic view of pelvis as seen during robotic laparoscopic procedure.

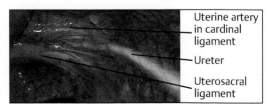

Fig. 11.3 Course and relation of ureter, uterosacral ligament, and uterine artery as seen laparoscopically.

Recognition of Ureteric Injury

About 62% of iatrogenic ureteral injury during hysterectomy goes unrecognized. This is more so with laparoscopic and robotic hysterectomy than open surgery. Therefore, a high degree of vigilance is required during laparoscopic and robotic hysterectomy to avoid missed iatrogenic ureteric injury.[16] The most common location of ureteric injury during gynecologic surgery is the lower one-third of ureter.[13] In large infiltrating pelvic tumors, middle third portion of ureter may be encased or invaded by tumor and is vulnerable to injury. But such large gynecologic tumors are rarely operated robotically. It is because (a) there is a limitation of space for the movement of instrument, (b) manipulation of such large tumor is nearly impossible by minimal invasive methods, and (c) there is no added advantage of minimal access surgery as a large incision will be required invariably for retrieval of specimen. Ureteric injury may be in the form of total or partial ligation by suture or clip, partial or complete transection with or without loss of a segment of ureter, thermal injury by monopolar or bipolar cautery, crushing, or hematoma.[17] A direct visualization of ureteric injury may rarely be encountered intraoperatively until searched vigilantly. An unrecognized ureteric injury significantly increases the readmission rate and may contribute to significant morbidity like the need for nephrostomy placement and urinary fistula. It may also cause potentially life-threatening complications like acute renal insufficiency, sepsis.[1]

Types of Ureteric Injury

- Ligation by suture or clip.
- Hematoma.
- Crushing by robotic instrument.
- Laceration.
- Partial or complete transection.
- Resection of ureter.
- Thermal injury by monopolar or bipolar cautery.

When to Suspect Ureteral Injury Intraoperatively

Most gynecologists do not encounter ureter during simple hysterectomy as they try to operate and dissect away from ureter and the ureter doesn't come in the way although it is in close vicinity of ureter. It is always better to identify and isolate ureter in difficult cases. The possibility of ureteric injury should be ruled out when dealing with adhesions, bulky uterus, or tumor with indistinct boundary. It should also be suspected when sutures or clips have been applied blindly or the operative field is messy at the presumed location of ureter after dissection. Pooling of urine in the operative field is rarely appreciable and is indicative of ureteric or bladder injury.

Intraoperative Recognition

One of the ways of identifying ureteric injury is to do endoscopic evaluation. It may be done by cystoscopy and by observing the jet of urine from the ureteric orifice.[18] Visualization of urinary jet may be enhanced by the use of intravenous injection of vital dyes like methylene blue or indigo carmine. However, the use of these vital dyes is not always without risk. Patients on serotonin reuptake inhibitors (Paroxetine, Fluoxetine, Sertraline, Citalopram, and Imipramine) may have serious serotonin toxicity after IV methylene blue.[19] Retrograde pyelogram (RGP) using radiocontrast and fluoroscope or retrograde injection of methylene blue can also be done to diagnose the ureteric injury and its location. But it is unpractical to do endoscopic evaluation while performing a robotic gynecologic surgery because it will require undocking of robotic arms, change of position from exaggerated lithotomy position to normal lithotomy position, and finally, it will invariably require positioning back again to exaggerated lithotomy or supine position for repair, in case an injury is detected which is not manageable endoscopically. In addition, a very different set of equipment like endoscope, irrigant, and C-arm needs to be available in the operating room. It also requires calling of an urologist because many gynecologists may not be well-versed in dealing with such complex issues.

Moreover, it causes increased operating and anesthesia time, which has its own consequences and cost associated. Furthermore, a suture partially occluding the ureteric lumen may be missed on RGP.[20] Hence, the role of universal cystoscopy for detection of ureteral injury is questioned. Most authors suggest that cystoscopy should be done in select cases.[21,22]

A more practical approach rather would be dissecting the ureter with robotic instruments only while patient is still in an exaggerated position after completion of gynecologic part of surgery.[23] Ureter is relatively easily identified as a tubular structure with a net of blood vessels woven around it and having peristalsis at a frequency of three to five per minute. Searching the ureter directly in the operative field may be difficult in patients with previous pelvic surgery, extensive adhesions due to endometriosis, or obscured operative field immediately after hysterectomy caused by charred tissue or excessive blood staining of tissue. In such cases, ureter may be traced antegrade after opening the overlying peritoneum well above the iliac vessels where still no dissection has taken place. The ureter can be easily traced by reflecting the caecum and ascending colon on the right side and sigmoid colon on the left side after incising the white line of Toldt. Here, one may get confused with another tubular structure running parallel to the ureter, (i.e., ovarian vein). However, it can be easily distinguished from the ureter, as it is relatively thin, bluish, and without peristalsis. Care should be taken not to peel off periureteral adventitial tissue while dissecting the ureter. The ureter gets its blood supply from multiple levels. The abdominal part receives multiple arterial branches from aorta located medially, and in the pelvic cavity blood vessels approach the ureter from laterally located iliac vessels and their branches. Hence, peritoneal covering should be opened laterally in the retroperitoneum and medially in the pelvic cavity.[10,11] While tracing the ureter antegrade, suspensory ligament of ovary and round ligament come in the way in cases where it had been preserved, such as simple hysterectomy. If it creates hindrance in perusing the ureter, it can be either divided or rolled back.

How to Avoid Ureteric Injury

Key to avoiding ureteric injury during robotic gynecologic surgery is the sound knowledge of anatomy of pelvis. The best way to prevent ureteric injury is to meticulously dissect the tissue in the pelvic cavity, and identify and isolate the ureter. Course of ureter and its relation with cervix, uterosacral ligament, cardinal ligament, gonadal vessel, and uterine artery should be born in mind while operating. Careful dissection of tissue plane should be done with identification

of individual structures like ureter and uterine artery. Many a time, individual structures are not identifiable. In such circumstances, one should stay close to cervix while severing the uterine artery or incising the vaginal cuff. The role of prophylactic placement of ureteral stent preoperatively in preventing ureteral injury and its cost-effectiveness is controversial.[24,25] Bilateral ureteral stenting can have its complications like anuria (1–5%), urinary tract infection, dysuria, and iatrogenic ureteric injury during stent placement (1%).[26–28] Moreover, ureteral stenting may fail in case of malignant ureteral involvement. Likewise, the use of light-emitting ureteral stent has also not conclusively proven beneficial in preventing ureteral injury.[29] One major limitation of robotic surgery is the lack of haptic feedback, which might help identify stented ureter as in open surgery and to a limited extent in laparoscopic surgery.

Management of Ureteric Injury

Timing of Repair

An intraoperatively discovered ureteric injury should be repaired immediately, although it does not ensure success, and many patients may develop urinoma and urinary fistula in the postoperative period.[30,31] Timing of postoperatively discovered ureteric injury remains debatable. An injury discovered within 3 days can be repaired immediately as an inflammatory response has not yet set in. An injury discovered after 72 hours should be repaired preferably after 6 weeks, but cure rates are similar to those repaired within 6 weeks.[23,32]

The intraoperative management of ureteric injury depends upon the site of injury, its length, and mechanism of injury. The most common site of ureteric injury during gynecologic surgery is in the lower third of the ureter. It may be partial or complete ligation by suture, metallic or Hem-O-lock clip, thermal injury, hematoma, laceration, or transection. The optimal way of managing this type of ureteric injury is ureteric reimplantation with or without psoas hitch and Boari flap reconstruction. For midureteric injury, ureteroureterostomy or transureteroureterostomy is an appropriate option. All these can be accomplished robotically or by open surgery.

The repaired ureteric injury should always be stented.

Principles of Managing Ureteric Injury

The golden principles of repair ureter include:
- Mobilize the ureter sparing adventitia.
- Debride the ureter until edges bleed, especially in thermal injury.
- Do spatulate, tension-free, watertight anastomosis over stent with absorbable fine sutures.
- Do retroperitonealization or omental wrapping wherever possible and place a drain.
- If immediate repair is not possible, do damage control by tying off the ureter with a long silk (for later identification and repair) and intraoperative (single J stent brought out cutaneously) or postoperative urinary diversion (percutaneous nephrostomy).[10,11]

Lower Ureteric Injury

A suture or clip should be removed and the viability of ureter is checked. In case of doubtful viability, it is better to resect the injured segment and do ureterourerostomy after careful mobilization of ureter to ensure a tension-free, spatulated anastomosis. A partial or complete transection and ureteral resection of <2 cm can also be managed by simple ureterourerostomy over a DJ stent.

When the defect in the ureter is more than 2 to 3 cm, a simple ureterourerostomy is not a wise option as limited mobilization may not confer tension-free anastomosis. In contrast, extensive mobilization can jeopardize the vascularity of ureter. The distal ureter is particularly vulnerable in this regard because of its tenacious blood supply.[33] In such cases, actual management depends on how distant the proximal healthy ureter's distal end is from the ureterovesical (UV) junction (**Table 11.1**). The distal ureter, however long, is not usable, and it should be closed.

In general, lower ureteric injury > 2 to 3 cm at any site from the crossing of iliac vessel to the bladder's entrance is manageable by ureteroneocystostomy (ureteric reimplantation) with or without psoas hitch and Boari flap (**Figs. 11.4** to **11.6**). Ureteroneocystostomy can be executed in refluxing or nonrefluxing manner and there is no significant difference in outcome.[34] Psoas hitch serves two purposes. It provides support to the anastomosis and brings bladder closer to

Table 11.1 Management of ureteric defects depending upon their length

Technique	Ureteral defect length (cm)
Ureteroureterostomy	2–3
Ureteroneocystostomy	4–5
Psoas hitch	6–10
Boari flap	12–15
Renal descensus	5–8

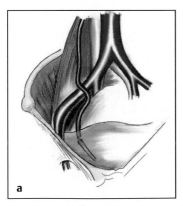 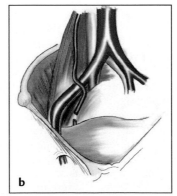 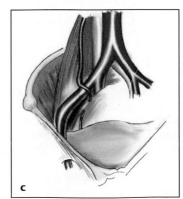

Fig. 11.4   Ureteric injury: Near ureterovesical junction (**a, b**), at crossing of iliac vessel (**c**).

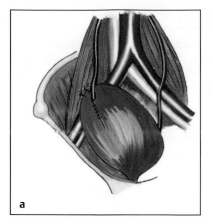

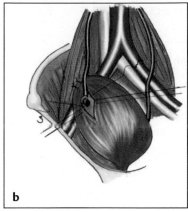

Fig. 11.5 (a, b) Uretero-neocystostomy with psoas hitch.

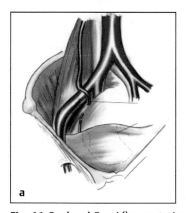

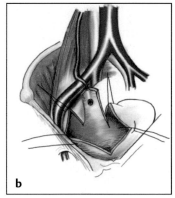

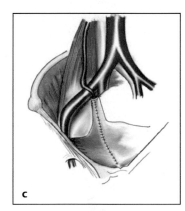

Fig. 11.6 (a–c) Boari flap ureteric reconstruction.

proximal segment of ureter so that a tension-free anastomosis can be facilitated. With psoas hitch, a gap of 6 to 10 cm between proximal ureteric stump and bladder can be bridged. One may require bladder mobilization and division of contralateral superior vesicle pedicle for hitching the bladder properly to psoas. One must be cautious while doing psoas hitch, as two important nerves are liable to get injured by this procedure. These are genitofemoral nerve which runs over the psoas major muscle and the femoral nerve running in the substance of psoas major muscle. Psoas hitch should be done over the psoas minor tendon or psoas major muscle.[35] Three to five interrupted absorbable 3–0 suture can be employed for this purpose. A larger defect where the stump of proximal ureter is at or above the pelvic brim (crossing of iliac vessel) and psoas

hitch does not ensure a tension-free anastomosis can be bridged by Boari flap.

Mid and Upper Ureteral Injury

A short midureteric injury (<2 cm) can be managed by ureteroureterostomy. Management of a large defect is challenging. It involves Boari flap ureteric reconstruction, transureterostomy, renal descensus, autotransplantation, Monti procedure, and ileal ureteral transposition. If intraoperative status of patient permits, the repair can be accomplished in the same sitting; otherwise, a damage control by closing the distal end of the proximal segment of ureter with a long nonabsorbable suture for later identification and urinary diversion by cutaneous ureterostomy or nephrostomy should be followed.[10,11]

Consequence of Unrecognized Ureteric Injury

The clinical presentation of an unrecognized ureteric injury depends upon the extant and mechanism of injury. A suture passing partially through the ureter can cause partial stricture and obstruction of ureter and resultant hydroureteronephrosis. It may be asymptomatic or cause dull aching pain. An occlusive suture can present in the postoperative period with severe pain in the flank, fever, and leukocytosis. An unrecognized lacerative ureteric injury or transection can result in the ureterovaginal fistula or urinary ascites. A thermal injury or devascularization injury can also present with delayed occurrence of ureterovaginal fistula or stricture. A patient with ureterovaginal fistula presents with continuous urinary leak with normal interval voiding. All such cases must be evaluated with computed tomography (CT) urography or intravenous urogram. Urological consultation should be sought for the management of all such cases. Initial management may be done with percutaneous nephrostomy in an attempt to make the patient dry, although this strategy may not always be successful. Expectant management with DJ stenting for 6 to 8 weeks can be done for partial ureteric stricture, but it usually fails. Further management depends upon the site and length of ureteric stricture or obstruction.[10,11]

Conclusion

The ureter is a vital structure in the gynecologic surgical field and liable to be injured, particularly during complex robotic surgery. A high degree of vigilance is necessary to avoid its injury and save the patient from suffering annoying postoperative morbidity. A recognized intraoperative injury can be safely and effectively repaired robotically.

Acknowledgments

Dr. Siddarth Kumar (senior resident, MCh, Urology, AIIMS Rishikesh) and Dr. Apurva Bariar provided all diagrams.

References

1. Blackwell RH, Kirshenbaum EJ, Shah AS, Kuo PC, Gupta GN, Turk TMT. Complications of recognized and unrecognized iatrogenic ureteral injury at time of hysterectomy: a population based analysis. J Urol 2018;199(6): 1540–1545

2. Abboudi H, Ahmed K, Royle J, Khan MS, Dasgupta P, N'Dow J. Ureteric injury: a challenging condition to diagnose and manage. Nat Rev Urol 2013;10(2):108–115

3. Williams PL, Bannister LH, Berry MM, et al. Gray's anatomy. 38th ed. New York: Churchill Livingstone; 1995

4. Drake RL, Vogl W, Mitchell AWM. Gray's anatomy for students. Philadelphia: Churchill Livingstone; 2005

5. Fröber R. Surgical anatomy of the ureter. BJU Int 2007;100(4):949–965

6. Hinman F, Stempen PH. Atlas of urosurgical anatomy. Philadelphia: WB Saunders; 1993

7. Moore KL, Dalley AF, Agur AM. Clinically oriented anatomy. 6th ed. Philadelphia: Lippincott Williams & Wilkins; 2010:292–365

8. Netter FH. Atlas of human anatomy. 5th ed. Philadelphia: Saunders; 2010

9. Eid S, Iwanaga J, Oskouian RJ, Loukas M, Tubbs RS. Comprehensive review of the cardinal ligament. Cureus 2018;10(6):e2846

10. Richard A, Santucci RA, Chen ML. Upper urinary tract trauma. In: Wein IJ, Kavoussi LR, Partin AW, Peters CA, eds. Campbell-Walsh urology. 11th ed. Philadelphia: Elsevier; 2016: 1158–1167

11. Nakada SY, Best SL. Management of upper urinary tract obstruction. In: Wein IJ, Kavoussi LR, Partin AW, Peters CA, eds. Campbell-Walsh urology. 11th ed. Philadelphia: Elsevier; 2016: 1133–1141

12. Manoel AGG, Anschau F, Gonçalves DM, Chrystiane da Silva M. Ureter: how to avoid injuries in various hysterectomy techniques, hysterectomy, Ayman Al-Hendy and Mohamed Sabry, IntechOpen doi:10.5772/30703. https://www.intechopen.com/books/hysterectomy/ureter-how-to-avoid-lesions-in-various-hysterectomy-techniques

13. Manoucheri E, Cohen SL, Sandberg EM, Kibel AS, Einarsson J. Ureteral injury in laparoscopic gynecologic surgery. Rev Obstet Gynecol 2012;5(2):106–111

14. Kiran A, Hilton P, Cromwell DA. The risk of ureteric injury associated with hysterectomy:

a 10-year retrospective cohort study. BJOG 2016;123(7):1184–1191

15. Park JH, Park JW, Song K, Jo MK. Ureteral injury in gynecologic surgery: a 5-year review in a community hospital. Korean J Urol 2012; 53(2):120–125

16. Parpala-Spårman T, Paananen I, Santala M, Ohtonen P, Hellström P. Increasing numbers of ureteric injuries after the introduction of laparoscopic surgery. Scand J Urol Nephrol 2008;42(5):422–427

17. Engelsgjerd JS, LaGrange CA. Ureteral injury. [Updated May 30, 2020]. In: StatPearls [Internet]. Treasure Island, FL: StatPearls Publishing; 2020. https://www.ncbi.nlm.nih.gov/books/NBK507817/

18. Vakili B, Chesson RR, Kyle BL, et al. The incidence of urinary tract injury during hysterectomy: a prospective analysis based on universal cystoscopy. Am J Obstet Gynecol 2005;192(5):1599–1604

19. Jeon HJ, Yoon JS, Cho SS, Kang KO. Indigo carmine-induced hypotension in patients undergoing general anaesthesia. Singapore Med J 2012;53(3):e57–e59

20. Morozov VV, Murphy L. Cystoscopy at the time of hysterectomy: does it make a difference? Austin J Obstet Gynecol. 2015;2: 1036. ISSN: 2378–1386

21. Sandberg EM, Cohen SL, Hurwitz S, Einarsson JI. Utility of cystoscopy during hysterectomy. Obstet Gynecol 2012;120(6):1363–1370

22. Advancing Minimally Invasive Gynecology Worldwide AAGL; AAGL Advancing Minimally Invasive Gynecology Worldwide. AAGL Practice Report: Practice guidelines for intraoperative cystoscopy in laparoscopic hysterectomy. J Minim Invasive Gynecol 2012;19(4):407–411

23. Liapis A, Bakas P, Giannopoulos V, Creatsas G. Ureteral injuries during gynecological surgery. Int Urogynecol J Pelvic Floor Dysfunct 2001;12(6):391–393, discussion 394

24. Schimpf MO, Gottenger EE, Wagner JR. Universal ureteral stent placement at hysterectomy to identify ureteral injury: a decision analysis. BJOG 2008;115(9):1151–1158

25. Kuno K, Menzin A, Kauder HH, Sison C, Gal D. Prophylactic ureteral catheterization in gynecologic surgery. Urology 1998;52(6):1004–1008

26. Merritt AJ, Zommere I, Slade RJ, Winter-Roach B. Oliguria after prophylactic ureteric stenting in gynaecological surgery—a report of three cases and review of the literature. Gynecol Surg 2014;11:23–26

27. Fugazzola P, Coccolini F, Tomasoni M, et al. Routine prophylactic ureteral stenting before cytoreductive surgery and hyperthermic intraperitoneal chemotherapy: safety and usefulness from a single-center experience. Turk J Urol 2019;45(5):372–376

28. Bothwell WN, Bleicher RJ, Dent TL. Prophylactic ureteral catheterization in colon surgery: a five-year review. Dis Colon Rectum 1994; 37(4):330–334

29. Redan JA, McCarus SD. Protect the ureters. JSLS 2009;13(2):139–141

30. Mandal AK, Sharma SK, Vaidyanathan S, Goswami AK. Ureterovaginal fistula: summary of 18 years' experience. Br J Urol 1990;65(5): 453–456

31. Grainger DA, Soderstrom RM, Schiff SF, Glickman MG, DeCherney AH, Diamond MP. Ureteral injuries at laparoscopy: insights into diagnosis, management, and prevention. Obstet Gynecol 1990;75(5):839–843

32. Brandt FT, Albuquerque CD, Lorenzato FR. Transperitoneal unstented ureteral reimplantation for injuries postgynecological surgery. World J Urol 2001;19(3):216–219

33. Michaels JP. Study of ureteral blood supply and its bearing on necrosis of the ureter following the Wertheim operation. Surg Gynecol Obstet 1948;86(1):36–44

34. Stefanović KB, Bukurov NS, Marinković JM. Non-antireflux versus antireflux ureteroneocystostomy in adults. Br J Urol 1991;67(3): 263–266

35. Brandes S, Coburn M, Armenakas N, McAninch J. Diagnosis and management of ureteric injury: an evidence-based analysis. BJU Int 2004;94(3):277–289

12 Robotic Radical Hysterectomy

Rajkumar Kottayasamy Seenivasagam and Karthik Chandra Vallam

Introduction

Radical hysterectomy (RH) requires significant technical skill and finesse with a steep learning curve even for the open procedure. The need for careful excision of parametrium with potential node-bearing lymphatics and lymph nodes and vaginal cuff while carefully preserving a vascularized ureter and innervations to the urinary bladder makes it a technically demanding procedure. While considering minimally invasive surgery (MIS) options, robotic surgery has advantages over laparoscopic dissection in providing finer and articulating instruments with increased dexterity, 3D vision, magnification, and a stable camera platform.[1] Challenges in RRH include longer operating time, steeper learning curve, loss of haptics, inability to change patient position intraoperatively, lesser choice of instruments, and the high costs involved in the surgery. Similar to robotic-assisted prostatectomy, robotic hysterectomy is likely to show significant advantages for patients, although evidence for the same is still awaited.

Indications and Evidence

Indications for robotic or robot-assisted radical hysterectomy (RRH) are similar to the open procedure (RH): Early stage cervical cancers (Stages IA1 with LVSI, IB1, IB2, IIA1, and some IB3/IIA2), cervical cancers with small central recurrence (<2 cm) postradiotherapy (RT) and endometrial cancers with cervical involvement or minimal parametrial involvement.[2,3] The type of RRH, type B or C (Querleu-Morrow),[4] is based on the stage of the disease, surgeons' expertise, and institutional practice. The authors' preference is type B for stage IA1 and IA2 and types C (C1/C2) for stage IB1, IB2, and IIA1. Bilateral pelvic lymphadenopathy (external and internal iliac) is typically done along with RRH. Some centers practice sentinel lymph node mapping in selected small (<2 cm) stage IA tumors with success.[5] Para-aortic lymphadenectomy (LND; below inferior mesenteric artery) is added in patients with advanced tumors or known pelvic nodal metastases.[3]

RRH has shown better early postoperative outcomes in reduced complications and shorter hospital stay[6–8] than open or laparoscopic RH. Though individual studies, both randomized and nonrandomized, showed equivalent or better survival results from RRH/MIS-RH compared to open RH,[9,10] the LACC trial[11] and a retrospective US National Cancer Database survey[12] showed inferior survival (both disease-free and overall) for MIS RH (including for RRH). Due to this, many societies across the world bring out guidelines against MIS RH and in favor of open RH.[13,14] However, the results of these studies should be accepted with caution.[14,15] Due to the steep learning curves involved in MIS RH, more robust evidence is required, and ongoing trials like RACC[16] may shed new evidence in this regard.

Anatomical Considerations

Preoperative Preparation

Preoperative evaluation and staging is usually done with an excellent pelvic examination and a contrast-enhanced CT (CECT) scan of the abdomen and pelvis. Some patients might require an examination under anesthesia or MRI pelvis for proper staging. Thorough preoperative anesthetic evaluation and reservation of blood for potential blood loss are essential. Many centers have adapted ERAS protocol for gynecologic surgeries.

The surgery is done under general and epidural anesthesia. The patient is placed in a steep Trendelenburg position with legs in Lloyd Davis straps. The anesthetist should be aware of this prior to surgery to plan for shoulder supports, extension lines for IV cannulas, arterial blood pressure monitors, etc., to avoid any interruptions or problems during the surgery. The bladder is drained using a 14-Fr Foley catheter. Second-generation cephalosporin is given as antibiotic prophylaxis. We do not use uterine manipulators but pack the vagina with betadine-soaked gauze roll.

Port Placement and Positioning

The technique described below is for a type C1 RRH performed on the da Vinci Xi platform (Intuitive Surgical Inc., USA). Pneumoperitoneum is established using a Veress needle. We use CO_2 pressures of 12 to 155 mmHg. The port configuration is shown in **Fig. 12.1**. The distance between pubic symphysis and camera (C) port should be 15 to 20 cm, and the distance between robotic (R1, R2, R3 ports) should be around 8 cm. Assistant (A) port is usually a 5-mm port and can be either placed in the right iliac fossa or the left hypochondrium. The port placement in the

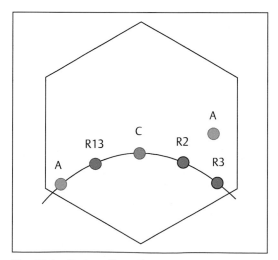

Fig. 12.1 Port configuration.

da Vinci Si platform (Intuitive Surgical Inc., USA) except for the R3 robotic port is not available. A diagnostic laparoscopy is done to rule out any peritoneal or liver metastases, to aid the release of adhesions, if any, and retract the small bowel and omentum away from the pelvis before the robot is docked oriented to the pelvis.

Camera targeting is done toward the uterus, and robotic instruments are docked into the arms. We commonly use monopolar scissors in R1, fenestrated bipolar forceps in R2, and ProGrasp forceps in R3 (all 8mm EndoWrist Instruments for da Vinci Xi platform).

Steps of the Procedure

The procedure follows the steps of open RH. The first step is the division of the round ligaments at the level of the lateral pelvic wall, followed by bilateral pelvic LND. By convention, we start with right-side pelvic LND. The anterior layer of the broad ligament (BL) is incised along the right lateral pelvic wall and the infundibulopelvic (IP) ligament is retracted superomedially to expose the right iliac vessels and right ureter crossing bifurcation of the right common iliac artery. The right ureter is also retracted medially along with the IP ligament, and LND is done systematically distal to proximal and lateral to medial, rolling the right external iliac artery and vein sequentially. It is essential to clearly define the boundaries of the dissection before LND: Laterally genitofemoral nerve, medially internal iliac artery, proximally common iliac bifurcation, distally deep inguinal ring, and posteriorly obturator nerve. The uterine dissected is the first medial branch of the internal iliac artery and is clipped and divided at the origin using Hemolok clips. The same steps are followed on the left side to address any adhesions at the descending-sigmoid colon junction. The nodes are placed into a specimen collection bag and left in the right iliac fossa. The 5-mm port may need to be converted into a 10- to 12-mm port to insert the collection bag.

Bilateral medial paravesical and pararectal spaces are defined using blunt dissection. Anteriorly, the bladder is dissected off the cervix and vagina using sharp dissection to gain a vaginal cuff margin of at least 2 cm. Ureters are dissected off the lateral parametrium (ureteric tunnel) using a combination of bipolar dissection and Hemolok clips preserving as much of the mesoureter as possible up to its entry into the bladder, thereby completely lateralizing the ureter.

Bilateral lateral parametrium is divided at the level of the internal iliac vessels except for the most caudal part to preserve the inferior hypogastric plexus. This resection is aided by lifting the ureter laterally and ventrally using a vascular sling or raising the mesoureter.

Ventral parametrium is resected at the level of the bladder after identifying and preserving the pelvic plexus nerves to the bladder. The rectouterine and rectovaginal ligaments are divided at the level of the rectum. This ultimately frees up the uterus except for the IP ligament and the vagina.

Bilateral IP ligaments are clipped and divided using Hemolok clips. We generally do not preserve the ovaries. The vaginal pack is now removed, and the vaginal cuff margins are assessed again. Vagina is resected with at least 2 cm margins all around. Uterine and LND specimens are retrieved per vaginally and vagina is closed using a V-loc suture.

Hemostasis is secured. We do not generally leave behind a pelvic drain. The port sites are closed with subcutaneous Vicryl and skin staplers. The procedure's total duration depends on the team's learning curve and is around 3.5 to 4 hours.

Tips and Tricks

- Leave the IP ligament intact till toward the end of the surgery. This provides an anchor for additional retraction.
- Use uterine artery clips to maneuver the parametrium and dissect off the ureter.
- Need to be patient, steady, and meticulous during dissection. The procedure has a steep learning curve.
- Don't hesitate to stent ureters preoperatively early in the learning curve or postoperatively in case of any doubt regarding vascularity.
- Dissect close to vessels and open up fascial planes clearly before proceeding to next step.

Postoperative Management

The Foley catheter is left in situ for 1 week and removed only after checking bladder sensation and urinary retention. Antibiotics are continued postoperatively for 5 to 7 days. We do not commonly use prophylactic LMWH, although it is recommended for pelvic cancer surgeries. The patient is started on a liquid diet the next day and slowly progressed to a normal diet before discharge. Normal postoperative stay is around 7 to 8 days, and the patient is discharged after removal of Foley's catheter.

Complications

Intraoperative complications include increased blood loss, ureter and bladder injuries, rectal injuries, nerve damage (genitofemoral, obturator, autonomic plexus) commonly due to thermal injury. Postoperative complications include infections (chest, pelvic, urinary), prolonged catheterization beyond 3 weeks, vaginal dehiscence, ureteric stenosis (due to thermal injury or decreased vascularity), prolonged hospitalization, port site hernia, and deep vein thrombosis. As mentioned earlier, RRH has better postoperative outcomes than open RH, including 1 to 2-day shorter hospital stay.

References

1. Renato S, Mohamed M, Serena S, et al. Robot-assisted radical hysterectomy for cervical cancer: review of surgical and oncological outcomes. ISRN Obstet Gynecol 2011;2011: 872434
2. National Comprehensive Cancer Network (NCCN). NCCN clinical practice guidelines in oncology. Uterine neoplasms, Version 1. NCCN; 2020. Retrieved from https://www.nccn.org/ professionals/physician_gls/pdf/uterine.pdf
3. National Comprehensive Cancer Network (NCCN). NCCN clinical practice guidelines in oncology. Cervical cancer, Version 1. NCCN; 2020. Retrieved from https://www.nccn.org/ professionals/physician_gls/pdf/cervical.pdf

4. Querleu D, Cibula D, Abu-Rustum NR. 2017 Update on the Querleu-Morrow classification of radical hysterectomy. Ann Surg Oncol 2017;24(11):3406–3412

5. Kadkhodayan S, Hasanzadeh M, Treglia G, et al. Sentinel node biopsy for lymph nodal staging of uterine cervix cancer: a systematic review and meta-analysis of the pertinent literature. Eur J Surg Oncol 2015;41(1):1–20

6. Park DA, Yun JE, Kim SW, Lee SH. Surgical and clinical safety and effectiveness of robot-assisted laparoscopic hysterectomy compared to conventional laparoscopy and laparotomy for cervical cancer: a systematic review and meta-analysis. Eur J Surg Oncol 2017;43(6):994–1002

7. Shazly SA, Murad MH, Dowdy SC, Gostout BS, Famuyide AO. Robotic radical hysterectomy in early stage cervical cancer: a systematic review and meta-analysis. Gynecol Oncol 2015;138(2):457–471

8. Roh HF, Nam SH, Kim JM. Robot-assisted laparoscopic surgery versus conventional laparoscopic surgery in randomized controlled trials: A systematic review and meta-analysis. PLoS One 2018;13(1):e0191628

9. Cantrell LA, Mendivil A, Gehrig PA, Boggess JF. Survival outcomes for women undergoing type III robotic radical hysterectomy for cervical cancer: a 3-year experience. Gynecol Oncol 2010;117(2):260–265

10. Mendivil AA, Rettenmaier MA, Abaid LN, et al. Survival rate comparisons amongst cervical cancer patients treated with an open, robotic-assisted or laparoscopic radical hysterectomy: a five year experience. Surg Oncol 2016;25(1):66–71

11. Ramirez PT, Frumovitz M, Pareja R, et al. Minimally invasive versus abdominal radical hysterectomy for cervical cancer. N Engl J Med 2018;379(20):1895–1904

12. Melamed A, Margul DJ, Chen L, et al. Survival after minimally invasive radical hysterectomy for early-stage cervical cancer. N Engl J Med 2018;379(20):1905–1914

13. Melamed A, Rauh-Hain JA, Ramirez PT. Minimally invasive radical hysterectomy for cervical cancer: when adoption of a novel treatment precedes prospective, randomized evidence. J Clin Oncol 2019;37(33):3069–3074

14. Rao ST, Nusrath S, Iyer R, et al. Interpretation and implications of LACC trial. Indian J Gynecol Oncolog 2019;17:39

15. Park JY, Nam JH. How should gynecologic oncologists react to the unexpected results of LACC trial? J Gynecol Oncol 2018;29(4):e74

16. Falconer H, Palsdottir K, Stalberg K, et al. Robot-assisted approach to cervical cancer (RACC): an international multi-center, open-label randomized controlled trial. Int J Gynecol Cancer 2019;29(6):1072–1076

13 Complications of Robotic Gynecologic Surgeries

Amit Gupta and Utkarsh Kumar

Abstract

Robotic surgery is increasing exponentially not only in gynecology but also in urological and abdominal surgeries. Surgeons should be skilled enough for open and laparoscopic approaches before performing robotic surgery so that untoward complications can be managed optimally. Nowadays, robotic systems are extending their arms in various procedures of gynecology for hysterectomy, sacrocolpopexy, myomectomy, adnexal surgery, and also in malignancies. The newer technology in the initial stages, with naïve surgeon skills, can lead to inadvertent complications, which can be minimized with proper knowledge on possible mishappenings reported in the literature. In this chapter, the authors have described different complications and their management in robotic gynecologic surgeries.

Introduction

United States Food and Drug Administration (USFDA) in 2005 approved the da Vinci robotic system in the field of gynecology. The da Vinci surgical system, in the past decade, has gained popularity for intricate gynecologic surgeries. The advantages of robotic surgery over laparoscopy are a greater degree of movement, precise dissection, 3D vision, tremor filtration, and a shorter learning curve. The other added advantages are decreased blood loss, quicker recovery, reduced hospital stay, less pain, and better cosmetic outcomes. In contrast to laparoscopic surgery, the disadvantages of robotic surgery are that it provides a fixed, stable field of vision, has high cost, and has lack of tactile sensation.

Conversion to open is one of the problems faced by surgeons during minimal access procedures, but conversion to open is not a failure but it is always wiser in difficult circumstances to prevent inadvertent disasters. The newer horizons in the field of robotics help the surgeons in exploring their use in complex and inaccessible pelvic surgeries. Its use is not only restricted to benign conditions but also is utilized in malignancies. In this chapter, the focus is on complications and management of robotic gynecologic surgeries.

Robotic Surgical Procedures and Complications

Benign

- Hysterectomy: Infection, hemorrhage, vaginal vault prolapses, injury to the ureter, bowel, or bladder, vesicovaginal fistula, venous thromboembolic events, and nerve injury are the complications of hysterectomy.
- Myomectomy: Complications are excessive blood loss, myometrial hematoma, and morcellation accident, bladder, bowel, fallopian injury, scarring, and infection.
- Sacrocolpopexy: Hemorrhage, urinary infection, febrile morbidity, wound infection, wound dehiscence, Ileus, etc., are the complications.
- Other robotic gynecologic surgeries: Pelvic organ prolapse, robotic surgery for endometriosis, robotic tubal anastomosis, robotic cerclage, prophylactic bilateral salpingo-oophorectomy, and robotic management of ectopic pregnancy. Robotic repair of posthysterectomy vaginal vault prolapses.

Malignancy

Robotic radical hysterectomy for cervical and uterine malignancies with pelvic and para-aortic lymphadenectomy.

Complications

As we know, the basic principles of laparoscopic and robotic surgery are the same. Therefore, prior trained laparoscopic surgeons with preoperative planning, intraoperative management, and post-operative follow-up can minimize complications.

Complications during Trocar Insertion

More than 50% of the complications (57%) are associated with trocar entry.[1] Body habitus, surgical history, gynecologic pathology, and surgeon's skills, prompt recognition, and adequate treatment are important. Umbilicus, sacral promontory, and bifurcation of major vessels are in the same alignment, so trocar injury chances are high. Early recognition by direct visualization of blood, hematoma, vital signs, and overlying bruise helps in identifying the vascular injury.

Jacobson et al found no substantial difference in complication rate based on the technique used.[2] Open Hasson's approach reduces vascular injury but not bowel injury;[3] it may reflect selection bias as Hasson's technique is used in high-risk patients (**Table 13.1**).

The following principles are used to reduce the incidence of trocar injury:

- The incision should be sufficient enough to allow trocar with mild force.

Table 13.1   Complication rates based on the technique of abdominal entry[2]

Technique	Complication rate per 1000
Direct trocar	0.6–1.1
Veress needle	0.3–2.7
Open laparoscopy	0.6–12.0
First trocar	1.9–2.7
Accessory trocar	0.8–6.0

- Prior catheterization should be done and the urinary bladder should be emptied.
- Use both hands during trocar insertion.
- Avoid Trendelenburg position during trocar insertion.
- Use the standard length of instruments and avoid long lengths (longer length only in morbidly obese patients).
- Avoid multiple punctures with a Veress needle.
- During insertion of trocar, increase abdominal pressure up to 15 mmHg for a short interval of time for maximum counter pressure.
- All secondary ports should be placed under direct vision.
- Inspect the first port entry site with a telescope for blood or any bowel content.
- Always check all the port entries and perform diagnostic laparoscopy before starting the actual procedure.
- Consideration of alternate access sites for the creation of pneumoperitoneum other than umbilicus in the previously operated abdomen.

Intraoperative Complications

Once assured that there is no injury during trocar insertion, the whole of the peritoneal cavity is inspected to assess pathology and distorted anatomy of pelvic organs, blood vessels, ureters, and bowel due to underlying pathology. Adhesiolysis and ureterolysis with the meticulous delineation of anatomy should be done. Correct identification of anatomical landmarks and pelvic structures decreases the risk of unintended injuries.

Complications Related to Electrical Energy

A major complication is electrical energy injury due to direct application, direct coupling, capacitive coupling, and sparking caused by defect in insulation. Understanding the biophysics of electrosurgery, tissue effect, knowledge of the equipment used, and types of injuries avoids electrical injury. Intraoperative identification of the mechanism of injury and its prompt management improves the postoperative outcomes.

Vascular Injury

These can be life-threatening injuries; most of these injuries are caused by Veress needle entry or by trocar but intraoperatively due to instrumentation or cautery (**Fig. 13.1**).

The bleeding from the abdominal wall from port site entry is mainly due to the inferior epigastric artery and can be recognized by continuous dribbling of blood from the trocar site or blood on the surface of the viscera and omentum. It can be controlled by direct pressure from the port, tamponade effect using Foley's as shown in **Fig. 13.2**, or by laparoscopic or open suture ligation. The major vascular injuries are managed as per the flowchart in **Fig. 13.3**.

Bowel Injury

Bowel injury is a catastrophic complication and can add significant morbidity and mortality if not recognized on time. Following standard surgical practices, meticulous dissection, and prompt recognition of bowel injury by a high index of suspicion are the key elements to prevent and manage potentially preventable disasters.

Most of the time, bowel perforation is not recognized at the time of surgery and can present as an acute abdomen in the postoperative period. The average time to diagnose small bowel injury by needle and cannula is 2 to 3 days and by electrocautery is 10 to 12 days. According to Toni Picerno et al, bowel injuries in robotic-gynecologic surgery are mostly colonic and rectal injuries. The overall incidence of bowel injury is 1 in 160 (0.62%; 95%; 0.50–0.76%). The type of surgical procedure did not make any significant differences in the incidence of bowel injury.[4]

If bowel injury is recognized on the table by fecal material from Veress needle or optical trocar and by direct visualization through the laparoscope, and if the injury is due to cold instruments and the size of perforation is very small, primary repair can be done robotically, laparoscopically, or by laparotomy depending upon the surgeon's skill and experience by standard single-layer extramucosal repair using 3.0 PDS. If there is electrosurgical damage or the size of perforation is large, consider segmental resection and reanastomosis or bowel diversion (ileostomy/colostomy) depending upon the site of perforation, hemodynamic stability, and biochemical parameter of patients.

Injury by Veress needle can be managed conservatively. Trocar injury is managed by leaving the trocar in place, identifying the site of trocar, and proceeding with laparotomy if the robotic approach is not feasible.

The presentation of bowel injury in the postoperative period may manifest initially as vague abdominal complaints, but most patients appear ill, and if the delayed presentation is pronounced, patients can become hemodynamically unstable. Prompt recognition by signs of peritonitis and the presence of intraperitoneal free air is detected by radiological investigation preferably CT scan with oral contrast. Although free air can be present in the postoperative period for 2 weeks after surgery, pneumoperitoneum on imaging should be taken as hollow viscus injury if clinical suspicion is high. The patient has to be resuscitated and should be taken for emergency exploratory laparotomy.

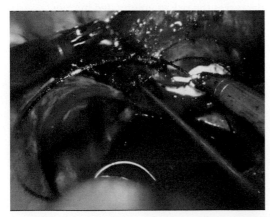

Fig. 13.1   Inadvertent spurter can obscure visual field.

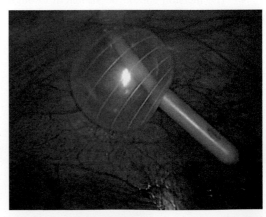

Fig. 13.2   Foley's tamponade to control abdominal wall bleed.

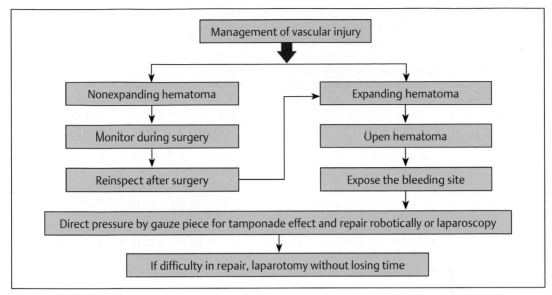

Fig. 13.3 Flowchart for management of vascular injury.

Genitourinary Tract Injury

It is one of the most common injuries with gynecologic surgery, especially during the hysterectomy. In laparoscopic hysterectomy, the urinary tract injury rate was 0.73%. According to procedure type, bladder and ureteral injury rates ranged from 0.05 to 0.66% and 0.02 to 0.4%, respectively.[5] Another study has shown urinary tract injuries were associated more with laparoscopic than an open abdominal hysterectomy (odds ratio 2.61; CI: 1.22-5.60).[6] The data on robotic procedures are lacking.

Urinary Bladder Injury

The urinary bladder injury is often secondary to suprapubic trocar placement in noncatheterized patients or during dissection of the pelvic region with a previous history of pelvic surgery or caesarean section. The urinary bladder can be found pulled up superiorly due to scarring. The location of bladder injury can be intraperitoneal or extraperitoneal and combined type.

The intraoperative detection and primary repair during the surgery have excellent results. Bladder injury is suspected if there is extravasation of urine (**Fig. 13.4**), visible laceration of the urinary bladder, clear fluid is visualized in the surgical field, bladder catheter, and blood or gas in urine bag during robotic/laparoscopic procedure.

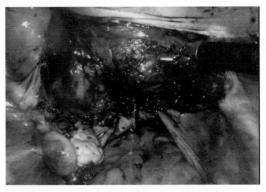

Fig. 13.4 Bladder injury: Iatrogenic bladder injury during robotic hysterectomy in a patient with history of previous two cesarean surgeries.

Large cystotomy is easily detected while smaller tears can be detected by instillation of methylene blue per urethral route. Cystoscopy is considered to localize the lesion in relation to the position of the trigone and ureteral orifices. If there is a lack of distension during cystoscopy, it is suggestive of a more extensive perforation. If detected intraoperatively, it can be managed with double-layer closure with Foley in situ for a week.

The postoperative bladder injury can be detected if there is increased abdominal distension, decreased urine output, and leakage from the vaginal cuff. If there is uncomplicated extraperitoneal injury, it can be managed conservatively with antibiotic prophylaxis and continuous bladder drainage with Foley's catheterization. The complicated extraperitoneal injury with symptomatic extravesical collection needs exploration, drainage, and repair. Intraperitoneal injuries need re-exploration with repair by double-layer closure using absorbable suture. Patients requiring operative repair for the urinary bladder injury should be kept on continuous Foley's catheter drainage followed by control cystogram and catheter removal after 14 days.

Ureteral Injury

The most common site of ureteral injury during robotic surgery is adjacent to uterosacral ligaments. The mechanism of ureteral injury is varied and often occurs due to ischemia caused by crushing with clamps, stripping of adventitia or thermal injury, transection (partial or complete) during dissection, and accidental ligature or clipping of ureters. The paramount way to prevent ureteral injury is by suitable operative approach, adequate exposure, avoiding blind clamping of blood vessels, direct visualization, and delineating the ureter and short diathermy applications. Preoperative prophylactic ureteral stenting aids in the visualization of ureters in complicated cases; however, it does not decrease the rate of injury. Routine use of cystoscopy does not seem to affect the detection rate of intraoperative lower urinary tract injury during robotic gynecologic surgery[7] (**Table 13.2**).

The management of ureteral injury depends on the nature, severity, length, and location of the injury. The optimal time to repair is during the surgery. The ligation injury can be managed by deligation and stent placement. Intraoperative partial ureter injury is best managed by robotic repair over Double J stent. In the case of complete transection, no tissue loss and distance of injury from vesicoureteral junction must be considered.

If the distance is less than 5 cm, ureteroneocystostomy should be considered, and if it is more than 5 cm, ureteroureterostomy. Similarly, various procedures have been described for complete ureteral transection depending on the extent of tissue loss like reimplantation of ureter using psoas hitch or Boari flap, transureteroureterostomy, replacement using ileal interposition graft, and renal autotransplantation in case of failed or multiple attempts of ureteral repair.

Erico Lustosa Ferreira et al observed ureterovaginal fistula (1.48%), vesicovaginal fistula (0.74%), and ischemia of the distal third of the ureter (0.74%) as early postoperative complications (**Table 13.3**).

Erico Lustosa Ferreira et al observed ureteral stenosis (2.96%), neurogenic bladder (1.48%), incisional bladder (1.48%), vesicovaginal fistula (0.74%), and incisional hernia with obstruction (0.74%) as late postoperative complications. Melamud et al in 2005 first reported the vesicovaginal fistula repair robotically (**Table 13.4**).

Vaginal cuff dehiscence is an early complication after hysterectomy.

Usually, the vaginal cuff is closed endoscopically in robotic-assisted surgery after uterus removal per vaginally but Uccella et al and Kho et al experienced the best results by two-layered transvaginal closure of the vaginal cuff.[8–10]

The advantages of performing this procedure are:
- The pneumoperitoneum does not need to be maintained.
- In the robotic surgical system, the needle holder is not required for the surgical procedure, which may decrease the costs for patients.
- The risk of vaginal cuff dehiscence is decreased.
- In the treatment of benign conditions, an assistant port is not required for the surgical procedure.

A randomized trial by Paraiso et al compared conventional and robotically assisted total

Table 13.2 Intraoperative complications during robotic gynecologic surgery[21-24]

Study	Bowel laceration/ injury	Ureteric laceration	Bladder injury	Vessels injury	Total
Ching-Hui Chen et al 2017	0.6%	0.1%	0.1%	–	0.8%
Ga Won Yim et al 2015	0.3%	–	0.3%	1.0%	1.6%
Erico Lustosa Ferreira et al	–	–	0.74%	–	0.74%

Table 13.3 Early postoperative complications after robotic gynecologic surgery

Study	Febrile morbidity	UTI	Ileus	Pelvic abscess	Vaginal cuff dehiscence/infection	Chylous ascites	Leg edema/weakness	Hematuria	Total
Ching-Hui Chen et al 2017	0.2%	1.2%	0.7%	1.8%	0.1%	-	-	-	4%
Ga Won Yim et al 2015	2.01%	0.33%	-	1.34%	2.68%	0.33%	2.01%	1.01%	14.4%
Erico Lustosa Ferreira et al	-	-	-	-	-	0.74%	-	-	3.7%

Table 13.4 Late postoperative complications

Study	Vaginal cuff dehiscence	Hydro-nephrosis	Wound infection	Ureterovaginal fistula	Voiding difficulty	Leg weakness	Peritonitis	Total
Ching-Hui Chen et al 2017	0.1%	0.2%	0.1%	0.2%	-	-	-	0.7%
Ga Won Yim et al 2015	-	0.33%	0.33%	0.33%	1.01%	0.33%	0.33%	2.7%
Erico Lustosa Ferreira et al	-	-	-	0.74%	-	-	-	11.8%

Table 13.5   Clavien-Dindo classification of postoperative complications

Study	I (no treatment)	II (need for pharmacological treatment)	III (intervention under anesthesia)	IV (intensive care due to single or multiorgan failure)	V (death)
Ching-Hui Chen et al 2017	0.9%	3.1%	6%	0.0%	0.0%
Ga Won Yim et al 2015	9.7%	5.4%	1.7%	0.0%	0.0%
Erico Lustosa Ferreira et al	4.44%	3.70%	8.14%	0.0%	0.0%

laparoscopic hysterectomy and reported 77 minutes less operating time for laparoscopic hysterectomy patients as compared to robotic but there was no difference in both groups in the occurrence of postoperative pain, complication rates, and duration of time to return to work.[11]

Patzkowsky et al compared the perioperative outcomes of hysterectomy performed by robotic and laparoscopic routes for benign diseases and identified that their conversion rate to laparotomy was lower in the robotic group as compared to the laparoscopy procedure (1.7% vs. 6.2%, $p=0.007$). However, the rates of urinary tract infection were higher in the robotic group. There were no differences in the rates of Clavien-Dindo grade I, grade II, and grade III surgical complications between these two groups (**Table 13.5**).[12]

Gobern et al reported that robotic-assisted laparoscopic myomectomies had longer operative times, but shorter hospital stays, less blood loss, and fewer transfusions than abdominal myomectomies. Robotic myomectomy offers a minimally invasive alternative for the management of symptomatic myoma.[13] Similar results were observed for sacrocolpopexy, adnexal surgeries, and endometriosis. The robotic surgeries had a longer duration of the procedure but there were no significant differences in relation to mean blood loss, hospital stay, and complication rates.[14–16]

A recent retrospective study compared hysterectomy with pelvic and para-aortic lymphadenectomy for endometrial carcinoma by robotic (n = 187) or laparoscopic (n = 245) methods. They found comparable rates of intraoperative complications (p = 0.525), but urinary injuries were higher in the laparoscopic group (p = 0.020). They also noted that patients in the robotic group had a shorter hospital stay (p = 0.016), but a mean operating time was 57 minutes more than the laparoscopic group which was statistically significant (p = 0.0001). There were no significant differences in blood transfusion rates and retrieval of the number of lymph nodes.[17]

Boggess et al compared open, laparoscopic, and robotic techniques for endometrial carcinoma and found that lymph node yield was higher for robotic techniques ($p<0.0001$) with lesser hospital stay ($p<0.0001$) and estimated blood loss ($p<0.0001$). Conversion rates were comparable in both groups. They concluded that staging by robotic technique is a feasible option and may be preferred. Ramirez et al did a retrospective study of stage IA cervical cancer patients who underwent robotic radical trachelectomy and bilateral lymphadenectomy and found that median operative time was 339.5 minutes (range 245–416 minutes) and median blood loss was 62.5 mL (range 50–75 mL), without intraoperative complications. No recurrences were observed at a median follow-up of 105 days. So, they interpreted that robotic is a safer procedure for cervix carcinoma.[18] Nick et al in 2012 observed similar results for stage IA and IB cervical cancer who underwent robotic radical trachelectomy and bilateral lymphadenectomy and the results were comparable with no recurrences.[19] Magrina et al compared laparoscopic, robotic, and open debulking surgery for ovarian cancer and found that the laparoscopy and robotic groups had similar perioperative outcomes.[20] The incidence of robotic system failure during surgery for robotic general surgical procedures and urologic and gynecologic surgeries has been reported to be 2.4 and 4.5%, respectively.

Conclusion

Finally, it can be concluded that the robotic system is safe and feasible not only for benign gynecologic diseases but also for gynecologic malignancies. With experience, the incidence of complications during surgeries can be minimized significantly. The authors strongly recommend regular practice on robotic simulators to decrease the overall incidence of complications.

References

1. Jansen F, Kapteyneyn K, Trimbos-Kemper T, Hermans J, Trimbos JB. Complications of laparoscopy: a prospective multi-center observational study. Br J Obstet Gynaecol 1997; 104:595–600
2. Jacobson MT, Osias J, Bizhang R, et al. The direct trocar technique: an alternative approach to abdominal entry for laparoscopy. JSLS 2002;6(2):169–174
3. Hasson HM. A modified instrument and method for laparoscopy. Am J Obstet Gynecol 1971;110(6):886–887
4. Picerno T, Sloan NL, Escobar P, Ramirez PT. Bowel injury in robotic gynecologic surgery: risk factors and management options. a systematic review. Am J Obstet Gynecol 2017; 216(1):10–26
5. Adelman MR, Bardsley TR, Sharp HT. Urinary tract injuries in laparoscopic hysterectomy: a systematic review. J Minim Invasive Gynecol 2014;21(4):558–566
6. Johnson N, Barlow D, Lethaby A, Tavender E, Curr L, Garry R. Methods of hysterectomy: systematic review and meta-analysis of randomised controlled trials. BMJ 2005; 330(7506):1478
7. Nguyen ML, Stevens E, LaFargue CJ, et al. Routine cystoscopy after robotic gynecologic oncology surgery. JSLS 2014;18(3): e2014.00261
8. Uccella S, Ghezzi F, Mariani A, et al. Vaginal cuff closure after minimally invasive hysterectomy: our experience and systematic review of the literature. Am J Obstet Gynecol 2011; 205(2):119.e1–119.e12. Back to cited text no. 31
9. Uccella S, Ceccaroni M, Cromi A, et al. Vaginal cuff dehiscence in a series of 12,398 hysterectomies: effect of different types of colpotomy and vaginal closure. Obstet Gynecol 2012;120(3):516–523
10. Kho RM, Akl MN, Cornella JL, Magtibay PM, Wechter ME, Magrina JF. Incidence and characteristics of patients with vaginal cuff dehiscence after robotic procedures. Obstet Gynecol 2009;114(2 Pt 1):231–235
11. Paraiso MF, Ridgeway B, Park AJ, et al. A randomized trial comparing conventional and robotically assisted total laparoscopic hysterectomy. Am J Obstet Gynecol 2013; 208(5):368.e1–368.e7
12. Patzkowsky KE, As-Sanie S, Smorgick N, Song AH, Advincula AP. Perioperative outcomes of robotic versus laparoscopic hysterectomy for benign disease. JSLS 2013;17(1):100–106
13. Gobern JM, Rosemeyer CJ, Barter JF, Steren AJ. Comparison of robotic, laparoscopic, and abdominal myomectomy in a community hospital. JSLS 2013;17(1):116–120
14. Paraiso MFR, Jelovsek JE, Frick A, Chen CCG, Barber MD. Laparoscopic compared with robotic sacrocolpopexy for vaginal prolapse: a randomized controlled trial. Obstet Gynecol 2011;118(5):1005–1013
15. Magrina JF, Espada M, Munoz R, Noble BN, Kho RMC. Robotic adnexectomy compared with laparoscopy for adnexal mass. Obstet Gynecol 2009;114(3):581–584
16. Nezhat C, Lewis M, Kotikela S, et al. Robotic versus standard laparoscopy for the treatment of endometriosis. Fertil Steril 2010;94(7): 2758–2760
17. Cardenas-Goicoechea J, Soto E, Chuang L, Gretz H, Randall TC. Integration of robotics into two established programs of minimally invasive surgery for endometrial cancer appears to decrease surgical complications. J Gynecol Oncol 2013;24(1):21–28
18. Ramirez PT, Schmeler KM, Malpica A, Soliman PT. Safety and feasibility of robotic radical trachelectomy in patients with early-stage cervical cancer. Gynecol Oncol 2010; 116(3):512–515
19. Nick AM, Frumovitz MM, Soliman PT, Schmeler KM, Ramirez PT. Fertility sparing surgery for treatment of early-stage cervical cancer: open vs. robotic radical trachelectomy. Gynecol Oncol 2012;124(2):276–280

20. Magrina JF, Zanagnolo V, Noble BN, Kho RM, Magtibay P. Robotic approach for ovarian cancer: perioperative and survival results and comparison with laparoscopy and laparotomy. Gynecol Oncol 2011;121(1):100–105

21. Chen CH, Chen HH, Liu WM. Complication reports for robotic surgery using three arms by a single surgeon at a single institution. J Minim Access Surg. 2017;13(1):22–28

22. Yim GW, Kim SW, Nam EJ, Kim S, Kim YT. Perioperative complications of robot-assisted laparoscopic surgery using three robotic arms at a single institution. Yonsei Med J. 2015;56(2): 474–481

23. Ferreira ÉL, Nunes JC, Zandoná M, Perret C, Fiorelli R, et al. Complications of robotic surgery in oncological gynecology: The experience of the Brazilian National Institute of Cancer. J Gynecol Res Obstet. 2019;5(2): 22–25

24. Melamud O, Eichel L, Turbow B, Shanberg A. Laparoscopic vesicovaginal fistula repair with robotic reconstruction. Urology. 2005;65(1): 163–166.

14 Robotics versus Laparoscopy for Gynecologic Surgery— The Evidence

Reeta Mahey and Monica Gupta

Introduction

The introduction of endoscopic surgery in gyne-cology has revolutionized women's health care. The main advantages of minimally invasive sur-geries (MIS) include better visualization, rapid postoperative recovery, shorter hospital stay, cosmetic benefits, and overall better patient satisfaction than laparotomy.[1] Almost all gyne-cologic surgeries, except advanced ovarian can-cers, can be done through a minimally invasive approach.

After years of utilizing standard laparoscopy (SL) in almost all types of gynecologic surger-ies, robotic-assisted laparoscopy (RAL) was introduced and approved by Food and Drug Administration (FDA) in 2005, with added bene-fits which are mainly wide range of movements comparable to human wrist, surgeons' comfort, possibility of minimizing surgeon tremors, and shorter learning curve as compared to conven-tional laparoscopy.[2] But even after 25 years since the inception of robotic surgery, it has not been able to justify its real benefit, especially for gyne-cologic surgery. The main reason for this is the overall high cost of the system and lack of haptic (tactile) feedback.[3]

The following questions need to be addressed during discussion of robotic versus laparoscopy for gynecologic surgeries:

1. Should we opt for robotic surgery over the laparoscopic route for all gynecologic surgeries?

2. What is the cost-benefit analysis of robotic versus laparoscopy for routine gyneco-logic surgeries?
3. Should we individualize and screen out which cases to be done by robotic route, and which can be managed through rou-tine laparoscopy?
4. What we need to teach our postgraduates and OBGYN residents?
5. How to counsel patients who enquire about the benefits of one route over the other?

Robot-assisted gynecologic surgery may be performed safely in centers with experienced surgeons. It has perioperative outcomes com-parable to laparoscopy and improved outcomes compared with laparotomy. Therefore, a min-imally invasive approach may be considered for procedures that might otherwise require laparotomy.[1] The real benefits of robotic-assisted surgery for gynecologic procedures are yet to be found for the cases where robotic route is said to be better than the laparoscopic route. It has been proven that MIS is better than laparotomy in terms of patient's satisfaction. But in terms of cost-effectiveness, MIS needs to be cheap and affordable. So we need to justify the cost that patient has to pay when offering a robotic route over a laparoscopy route.

Although robotic surgery has been proved beneficial in urological surgeries, its role in gynecologic surgery compared to tradi-tional laparoscopy is yet to be established.

Patients undergoing gynecologic procedures of short duration, especially of low complexity, are unlikely to benefit from robotic-assisted surgery. Due to lack of advantages and potential disadvantages, the American College of Obstetricians and Gynecologists (ACOG) and the Society of Gynecologic Surgeons (SGS) recommend not to use the robotic route for tubal ligation, ovarian cystectomy, ectopic pregnancy, salpingo-oophorectomy, and simple diagnostic laparoscopy.[1]

Comparison of RAL versus SL for Various Benign Gynecologic Surgeries

Hysterectomy

Worldwide, hysterectomy is the most common gynecologic surgery done for various indications. Both AAGL and ACOG have recommended using laparoscopic route for hysterectomy where vaginal route is not feasible. Some reports have been published on robot-assisted hysterectomy, but assessments of robotic surgery costs are complex and dependent on many factors, (e.g., usage and surgeon experience). No mean difference in operative time has been found in studies comparing robot-assisted hysterectomy with abdominal and laparoscopic approaches.[4] Vaginal cuff dehiscence and cuff complications have been reported to be less with intracorporeal suturing as compared to vaginal route for cuff closure.[5] But no difference has been documented between cuff complications when laparoscopic hysterectomy was compared to robot-assisted hysterectomy.[6]

Myomectomy

The evidence is also low for any added benefits of the robotic route for myomectomy as compared to the laparoscopic route. In a systematic review comparing robotic myomectomy with laparoscopic and open myomectomy, robot-assisted laparoscopic myomectomies had longer operative times compared with abdominal approaches. However, blood loss, rates of transfusion, and length of hospital stays were substantially reduced. Comparison with laparoscopic route reported 4.5 times higher conversion to

laparotomy in the laparoscopy route as compared to robotic route.[7] Prospective data is required on added advantage of RAL for myomectomy over conventional laparoscopy in terms of reproductive outcomes.

Endometriosis Surgery

RAL may be considered better for patients with deep infiltrating endometriosis (DIE), especially those involving bowel or urinary tract. But in the studies done as comparative studies between RAL and SL to manage endometriosis, no substantial advantages of RAL have been seen over SL. Even the studies reported significantly reduced operative time in patients operated by SL.[8,9] Because in these studies, the comparison between RAL and SL has been limited to perioperative outcomes, by no means has it been possible to draw any conclusion about the most important outcomes such as long-term relief of pain, pregnancy rates in infertile women, and improvement in quality of life. Only adequately designed randomized trials comparing RAL and SL for the treatment of endometriosis would disentangle these issues.

Sacrocolpopexy

As discussed with other gynecologic procedures, sacrocolpopexy has also shown better outcomes through robotic compared to open laparotomy route, but the studies comparing laparoscopy versus robotic route have not shown any benefits of the robotic route.[10]

RAL versus SL in Gynecologic Oncology

The most robust evidence of the role of RAL versus SL is in women with endometrial cancers. Several meta-analyses have shown lesser blood loss and lesser rates of conversion to laparotomy but comparable operative time, length of hospital stay, complications, and oncological outcome.[11] There is less consistent data in surgical management of cervical and early stage ovarian cancer, and RAL is not superior to SL.[12,13]

Netter et al have reported some benefits of RAL over SL for gynecologic cancer in patients with complex factors (elderly, high body mass index, procedures requiring lymphadenectomy) in terms of operating time and length of post-operative hospital stay.[14] The only consensus regarding surgical management of gynecologic cancers is that MIS is superior to open surgery for peri and early postoperative outcome but recently its role regarding long-term oncological outcomes is questioned, especially in early stage cervical cancer. Further prospective randomized studies are required to prove or disprove the actual benefits of RAL over SL in terms of immediate postoperative and long-term outcomes in gynecologic cancers.[15]

Choice of Route of Surgery

When choosing the route of surgery, individual patient characteristics and surgeon's expertise should be taken into account. ACOG issued a general evidence-based recommendation, "Choosing wisely," which stated to avoid using robotic route for benign gynecologic conditions and, wherever feasible, to use vaginal or conventional laparoscopic approach.[16] For women with DIE, laparoscopy is the minimally invasive route of choice. RAL has not shown any proven benefits over standard laparoscopy in women with endometriosis. So due to the high cost associated with RAL, the robotic route should be avoided outside the research settings.[17] Suppose the surgeon is experienced in managing severe endometriosis, and proper preoperative evaluation and mapping have been done with transvaginal sonography (TVS) and/or magnetic resonance imaging (MRI), in that case, SL provides a safe and cost-effective approach to manage these cases and role of RAL is yet to be justified.

Cost-Benefit Analysis

If we compare RAL and SL, the issue of costs is of paramount importance, as RAL technique is more expensive than the latter one. Expenses for RAL are related to the cost of around 2 million euros for the robot itself, the annual maintenance fee of around 160,000 euros, and the cost of 1200 to 2000 euros of each robotic instrument, which must be mandatorily replaced after ten surgical procedures.[18] Consequently, to justify widespread use of a more expensive technique (RAL),

the technique has to prove advantageous over SL with better outcomes for the patients.

Conversion to Laparotomy

Another point of discussion has been conversion to laparotomy. In women undergoing surgery for endometrial cancer, a low laparotomy conversion rate is seen with RAL as compared to SL.[11] Again, we need to justify while offering such expensive and sophisticated techniques that increase overall surgery-related expenses. According to the data available to date, RAL provides no extra benefit for surgeons already trained in SL techniques, at least in benign gynecologic surgeries.[1]

Operative Field

While debating for RAL over SL, operative field is an important parameter, especially when surgery is not limited to pelvis. In RAL, the camera is not interchangeable in-between the ports and movements of ports are also limited. To operate in a field away from pelvis, it becomes necessary to undock the robot in-between and complete the procedure through laparoscopy. This is in contrast to SL where the camera may be exchanged in-between the ports and movements of camera and accessary ports are accessible in all directions. A study evaluating colorectal resection in cases of endometriosis reported a significantly higher time of surgery in RAL compared to SL.[19] So, RAL does not justify its role in women with severe cases of endometriosis requiring surgery outside the pelvis and bowel resection.

Learning Curve

A comparatively shorter learning curve has been reported in minimally invasive suturing with robotic assistance than SL, especially for novice surgeons, but benefit is less clear among experienced ones.[20] Recent randomized studies have demonstrated similar learning curves and equivalent performance but have shown advantage of robotized instruments in ergonomically difficult conditions.[21]

Indian Scenario

In India and other low- and middle-income countries (LMIC), the overall cost of equipment and surgery is a significant factor. So, it is must to choose patients who are actually going to be benefitted from robotic route. We need more data to prove the actual benefits of robotic routes for most gynecologic surgeries considering cost as a significant factor and real gain over laparoscopic approach.

Till the cost of robot comes down to the affordable levels, it cannot be offered as a replacement of the laparoscopic route. Along with surgeon's interests, patient's choice and cost should be taken into account while deciding the surgery route.

Conclusion

Any new surgical technique should be adopted based on actual benefits to the patients, cost analysis, and evidence-based medicine rather than justifying the technique due to external pressure.[1] Robotic-assisted routes should be selected based on the likelihood of improved outcomes than other surgical approaches in terms of patient factors, cost factors, and complexity of the individual case. A patient going for robotic-assisted surgery should be informed about the actual benefits and risks associated with the robotic route and other available alternative surgical approaches.[1] The lack of sufficient level-1 evidence in the literature addressing robotic surgery underlies the inability to identify and delineate the benefits of robotics in benign gynecologic procedures, especially hysterectomy.[3]

As all the studies stating benefits of robotic route for gynecologic surgeries are retrospective and nonrandomized, we have yet to find the robotic route's real benefits, especially for benign gynecologic surgeries. Another important aspect and need are to take the overall cost of surgery into account when analyzing the real benefits of the robotic route. Randomized controlled trials or comparably rigorous nonrandomized prospective trials are the need of hour to determine the patient subgroup likely to benefit from robotic route surgery.

References

1. Robot-assisted surgery for noncancerous gynecologic conditions. ACOG Committee Opinion No. 810. American College of Obstetricians and Gynecologists. Obstet Gynecol 2020;136:e22–e30
2. Sinha R, Sanjay M, Rupa B, Kumari S. Robotic surgery in gynecology. J Minim Access Surg 2015;11(1):50–59
3. Madueke-Laveaux OS, Advincula AP. Robot-assisted laparoscopy in benign gynecology: advantageous device or controversial gimmick? Best Pract Res Clin Obstet Gynaecol 2017; 45:2–6
4. Sarlos D, Kots L, Stevanovic N, Schaer G. Robotic hysterectomy versus conventional laparoscopic hysterectomy: outcome and cost analyses of a matched case-control study. Eur J Obstet Gynecol Reprod Biol 2010;150(1):92–96
5. Uccella S, Malzoni M, Cromi A, et al. Laparoscopic vs transvaginal cuff closure after total laparoscopic hysterectomy: a randomized trial by the Italian Society of Gynecologic Endoscopy. Am J Obstet Gynecol 2018;218(5):500.e1–500.e13
6. Dauterive E, Morris G IV. Incidence and characteristics of vaginal cuff dehiscence in robotic-assisted and traditional total laparoscopic hysterectomy. J Robot Surg 2012; 6(2):149–154
7. Iavazzo C, Mamais I, Gkegkes ID. Robotic assisted vs laparoscopic and/or open myomectomy: systematic review and meta-analysis of the clinical evidence. Arch Gynecol Obstet 2016;294(1):5–17
8. Nezhat CR, Stevens A, Balassiano E, Soliemannjad R. Robotic-assisted laparoscopy versus conventional laparoscopy for the treatment of advanced stage endometriosis. J Minim Invasive Gynecol 2015;22(1):40–44
9. Nezhat FR, Sirota I. Perioperative outcomes of robotic assisted laparoscopic surgery versus conventional laparoscopy surgery for advanced-stage endometriosis. JSLS 2014; 18(4): e2014.00094
10. Li H, Sammon J, Roghmann F, et al. Utilization and perioperative outcomes of robotic vaginal vault suspension compared to abdominal or vaginal approaches for pelvic organ prolapse. Can Urol Assoc J 2014;8(3-4):100–106
11. Rabinovich A. Minimally invasive surgery for endometrial cancer. Curr Opin Obstet Gynecol 2015;27(4):302–307

12. Zhou J, Xiong BH, Ma L, Cheng Y, Huang W, Zhao L. Robotic vs laparoscopic radical hysterectomy for cervical cancer: a meta-analysis. Int J Med Robot 2016;12(1):145–154

13. Minig L, Padilla Iserte P, Zorrero C, Zanagnolo V. Robotic surgery in women with ovarian cancer: surgical technique and evidence of clinical outcomes. J Minim Invasive Gynecol 2016;23(3):309–316

14. Netter A, Jauffret C, Brun C, et al. Choosing the most appropriate minimally invasive approach to treat gynecologic cancers in the context of an enhanced recovery program: Insights from a comprehensive cancer center. PLoS One 2020;15(4):e0231793

15. Kerbage Y, Kakkos A, Kridelka F, et al. Lomboaortic lymphadenectomy in gynecological oncology: laparotomy, laparoscopy or robot-assisted laparoscopy? Ann Surg Oncol 2020;27(10):3891–3897

16. American College of Obstetricians and Gynecologists (ACOG). 2016. Choosing wisely. Ten things physicians and patients should question. Recommendation #6 revised August 24. https://www.acog.org/-/media/Departments/Patient-Safety-and-Quality-Improvement/Choosing-WiselyOct2016.pdf?dmc = 1 and ts = 20170201T1343323012

17. Berlanda N, Frattaruolo MP, Aimi G, et al. "Money for nothing." The role of robotic-assisted laparoscopy for the treatment of endometriosis. Reprod Biomed Online 2017;35(4):435–444

18. Paul S, McCulloch P, Sedrakyan A. Robotic surgery: revisiting "no innovation without evaluation". BMJ 2013;346:f1573

19. Cassini D, Cerullo G, Miccini M, Manoochehri F, Ercoli A, Baldazzi G. Robotic hybrid technique in rectal surgery for deep pelvic endometriosis. Surg Innov 2014;21(1):52–58

20. Møller SG, Dohrn N, Brisling SK, Larsen JCR, Klein M. Laparoscopic versus robotic-assisted suturing performance among novice surgeons: a blinded, cross-over study. Surg Laparosc Endosc Percutan Tech 2020;30(2):117–122

21. Siri E, Crochet P, Charavil A, Netter A, Resseguier N, Agostini A. Learning intracorporeal suture on pelvitrainer using a robotized versus conventional needle holder. J Surg Res 2020;251:85–93

15 Cost-Benefit Analysis of Robotic Gynecologic Surgery: Costly or Cost-Effective?

Anupama Bahadur, Anoosha K. Ravi, and Rajlaxmi Mundhra

Introduction

Since FDA approval in 2005, gynecologic surgeons all over the world have embraced this innovative new technology. Banking more and more hours at the console and mastering this skill has been very rewarding, as are the satisfied patients. But, what is it that it is offering over and above the already existing time-tested approaches like open, vaginal, and laparoscopic? Robotic technology was intended to overcome the drawbacks of laparoscopy in the minimally invasive field. But the evidence so far majorly reflects it as an expensive but equally effective alternative to laparoscopy.[1-4] So why choose robot over laparoscope? Is it only a costly affair or a cost-effective one?

Evidence so Far

The minimally invasive approach has been irrevocably proven to be better than the open method with lesser blood loss, lesser postoperative complications, better cosmesis, and faster return to routine activities.[5] So the fair comparison of the robotic approach is with that of laparoscopy and vaginal when applicable. Comparing these modalities is complicated by biases like the familiarity of older methods or reluctance to accept new, robotic is relatively newer and not widely available, lack of competition in robotic technology, insurance coverage, and study methodologies. A systematic review of studies conducted before May 2016 was done with Consolidated Health Economic Evaluation Reporting Standards (CHEERS) by Korsholm et al.[6] Among 32 studies which were included in the review, none of them fully complied with the checklist, and only three of them factored in the societal perspective of cost analysis. The flawed methodological designs of studies comparing the cost of different modalities can wrongly influence the decision-making.

Factors in Consideration

Many things influence the cost of a surgical modality:
- Initial investment and maintenance of equipment.
- Recurring cost per case:
  - Instruments.
  - Drapes.
- Operative variables:
  - Surgical team.
  - OT time.
  - Difficulty level.
- Postoperative recovery:
  - Blood transfusion.
  - Analgesic and antiemetic requirement.
  - Length of hospital stay.
  - Postoperative complications.
- Societal cost:
  - Loss of days off work.
  - Revisits to hospital.
  - Patient satisfaction.
- Training of residents.

The Initial Investment

The initial investment is one of the most crucial factors which outcasts robotic surgery as the most expensive modality. da Vinci robotic system has dominated unanimously for almost two decades in the field. This being the newest and latest technology without a competitor in the market is an unmodifiable expense at present. Like any new advancement, this is an expected occurrence in the surgical field. Decreased willingness to pay could significantly impact this factor, but too much time has elapsed since the debut for this to be a reality. With so many technologies in active research, it won't be too long before there is the competition to the price.[7] Willingness to pay has also been the reason why robotic surgeries have not been uniformly practiced.

The cost analysis study is primarily affected by the initial expense of robotic surgeries in comparison to laparoscopy or open methods. With that of laparoscopy, it is generally assumed as preexisting equipment and not accounted for. In a randomized trial comparing vaginal, laparoscopic, and robotic hysterectomy, the cost of robotic was comparable to laparoscopy when the robotic machine was considered a preexisting investment ($7059 vs. $7016).[4] Similar to laparoscopy, when the robotic machine is utilized by multiple surgical specialties, and in larger volume, fixed costs like initial investment and maintenance charges are less pronounced.

With increasing popularity among surgeons and patients for both benign and malignant indications, a more significant percentage of insurance coverage and reimbursement will also downsize the cost factor.

Recurring Cost

Recurring cost is due to robotic instruments, drapes, and ancillary equipment. Robotic instruments have a limit of 10 uses per instrument before it should be replaced. The number of uses is logged in the moment the particular instrument is docked. Robotic trocars and instruments are unique to da Vinci surgical system. Instrument costs range from $220 to $320 each per use.[8] In a robot-assisted hysterectomy, three arms with one for the camera, one for bipolar forceps, and one for monopolar scissors are mandatory. One can have two more arms with one each for prograsp and needle holder. Prograsp, unlike needle holder, is used throughout the surgery and very useful in complex cases with a large uterus, lymphadenectomy in a case of carcinoma, etc. A recent Indian study successfully demonstrated the safety and efficacy of using prograsp forceps in place of a needle holder for vaginal cuff closure, thus reducing the cost of one instrument.[8] With smaller uterus, uterine manipulator can be placed and prograsp can also be avoided. Uterine manipulators range from $29 ZUMI to $90 RUMI.[9] For entry into the peritoneum, two-step closed entry with Veress needle ($15) is the cheapest compared to open entry with Hasson ($50) or optical trocars.[9]

Another important cost-cutting solution would be to place an accessory port/assistant port for reusable laparoscopic instruments like myoma screw, suction irrigator, and retractor. Sterile disposable drapes used for robotic columns and arms contribute to the recurring cost. Whenever a robotic arm is not being used, one of the drapes can be saved for later use, thus minimizing the cost per case.

The skill of the robotic surgeon mimics open surgery but with a computerized interface. Hence, the learning curve has been shorter, unlike laparoscopy surgeries. Though shorter, studies earlier in the time since FDA approval in 2005 accounted robotic learning curve as an added cost as surgeons have already traversed the learning curves for laparoscopy and open.[10] The surgeon and the entire surgical team, including anesthetists, residents, technicians, and nursing staff, must be trained in robotic surgery for the operating room to work like a well-oiled machine.[11–13] It is believed that with increasing surgeon experience and dedicated surgical team, the operative variables like docking time, operative time, and specimen retrieval time can all be at their optimum. This has been observed in a multicenter analysis for different modes of hysterectomies by high-volume surgeons.[14,15] Thus consistency breeds efficiency, and efficiency reduces costs.

OT time is also affected by the difficulty level and extent of surgery. Larger uterine weights add to the complexity of surgery.[16,17] When this variable is factored in, robotic surgery is a more cost-effective modality compared to open and even laparoscopy. In a retrospective analysis by Moawad et al, with uterine weight >750 g, laparoscopic procedures added 47 minutes to operative time and $1648 to the cost.[18] Myomectomies are inherently a bloody procedure. With minimal invasive approaches like robotic or laparoscope, the blood loss and need for blood transfusion, intra and postoperative complications are minimal compared to open myomectomies.[5,19] This translates to lesser costs.

The obese subset of patients definitively benefits from robotic surgeries. It was one of the intended effects of robotic surgery over laparoscopy surgery. Despite higher body mass index (BMI), the conversion rates to laparotomy are significantly lower in robotic surgery than laparoscopic surgery.[20,21]

Among malignancies, endometrial cancer staging has been successfully realized with a minimal invasive approach. In the LAP2 study, a randomized control trial, laparoscopy was a safe-and-effective alternative to laparotomy with identical overall survival.[22] With lower conversion rates and better lymphadenectomy rates, robotic surgery has been equally cost-effective if not superior to laparoscopy.[23] In a single-institution study by Bell et al, blood loss and complication rates were significantly lower in the robotic group than in laparotomy. Returning to normal activity was faster than laparoscopy and laparotomy. The total average cost of robotic surgery was cheaper than laparotomy and 700 $ costlier than laparoscopy.[16]

A shorter hospital stay compensates for the added expense in the operating room in terms of machines and instruments. Several studies have observed a significantly lower hospital stay favoring robotic surgery.[21,24] With lesser antiemetics, analgesics wound complications, and adhesions, the rate of readmissions is also minimal with robotic surgery.[25,26]

There are three separate models in which cost comparison between different modalities is done; societal perspective model, hospital perspective model, and hospital perspective without robot costs model. But only the societal perspective model is a justified approach as it includes lost wages and caregiver cost, which play an essential role in overall costs. Barnett et al studied different modes of hysterectomy in endometrial cancer and found that robotic surgery is cheaper than abdominal and is the most economically attractive as disposable equipment costs are minimized.[27] In a randomized control trial comparing conventional laparoscopy with robotic hysterectomy, Sarlos et al found that the postoperative quality-of-life index was better with robotic surgeries; however, in the long-term there was no difference.[3] In a contradictory analysis by Jonsdottir et al the lowest indirect cost to society was found with robotic surgery compared to laparoscopic, abdominal, and vaginal hysterectomies.[28]

Cost of Residency Training

A resident is expected to be trained in all modalities, whether cost-effective or not. Though open surgeries have substantially reduced since the introduction of the minimal invasive approach, still a majority of them are being performed with laparotomy.[29] On contrary to popular belief, the introduction of robotics has rather increased the rate of laparoscopy surgery as reported by Knight et al[30] or has not decreased as reported by Wright et al.[1] But how well are residents getting trained in the robotic console? Since it is a new technology, there has been a lag in training of residents with that of surgeons as per several surveys.[31,32] But on the bright side, robotic surgery is here to stay, and training does not end with residency. Also with an increasing percentage of robotic surgeries, there is a hopeful expected rise in resident training.

With all this said, on any day, if the vaginal approach is applicable, it should always be preferred over robotic or laparoscopy or open surgery.[4,33,34]

Conclusion

Robotic surgeries in the field of gynecology, benign or malignant, are a cost-effective modality. It comes across as the most expensive technology, but a surgical system's cost does not end at the operating room. The benefit of shorter hospital stay, lesser postoperative complications, and faster recovery with robotic surgery offsets the cost of machines and instruments. With upcoming competitive systems to da Vinci surgical system, initial investment expense is also expected to get minimized. In the meanwhile, it is observed that with broader usage of robotic surgeries, the fixed costs like purchasing and maintenance costs are less pronounced. Robotic surgeries are rather more cost-effective than open or laparoscopy in cases with high BMI, dense adhesions, larger uterus, or need for lymphadenectomy.

References

1. Wright JD, Ananth CV, Lewin SN, et al. Robotically assisted vs laparoscopic hysterectomy among women with benign gynecologic disease. JAMA 2013;309(7):689–698
2. Paraiso MF, Ridgeway B, Park AJ, et al. A randomized trial comparing conventional and robotically assisted total laparoscopic hysterectomy. Am J Obstet Gynecol 2013; 208(5):368.e1–368.e7
3. Sarlos D, Kots L, Stevanovic N, von Felten S, Schär G. Robotic compared with conventional laparoscopic hysterectomy: a randomized controlled trial. Obstet Gynecol 2012; 120(3):604–611
4. Lonnerfors C, Reynisson P, Persson J. A randomized trial comparing vaginal and laparoscopic hysterectomy versus robot-assisted hysterectomy. J Minim Invasive Gynecol 2015;22:78–86
5. Iavazzo C, Mamais I, Gkegkes ID. Robotic assisted vs laparoscopic and/or open myomectomy: systematic review and meta-analysis of the clinical evidence. Arch Gynecol Obstet 2016;294(1):5–17
6. Korsholm M, Sørensen J, Mogensen O, Wu C, Karlsen K, Jensen PT. A systematic review about costing methodology in robotic surgery: evidence for low quality in most of the studies. Health Econ Rev 2018;8(1):21
7. Iavazzo C, Papadopoulou EK, Gkegkes ID. Cost assessment of robotics in gynecologic surgery: a systematic review. J Obstet Gynaecol Res 2014;40(11):2125–2134
8. Rajanbabu A, Patel VJ, Appukuttan A. Reducing the cost of robotic hysterectomy: assessing the safety and efficacy of using prograsp forceps in lieu of needle holder for vaginal cuff closure. J Robot Surg 2021;15(1):31–35
9. Sanfilippo SJ, Snook LM. Cost-conscious choices for minimally invasive gynecologic surgery. OBG Manag 2013;25(11):40–72
10. van Dam P, Hauspy J, Verkinderen L, et al. Are costs of robot-assisted surgery warranted for gynecological procedures? Obstet Gynecol Int 2011;2011:973830
11. Nash K, Feinglass J, Zei C, et al. Robotic-assisted laparoscopic myomectomy versus abdominal myomectomy: a comparative analysis of surgical outcomes and costs. Arch Gynecol Obstet 2012;285(2):435–440
12. Dimick JB, Chen SL, Taheri PA, Henderson WG, Khuri SF, Campbell DA Jr. Hospital costs associated with surgical complications: a report from the private-sector National Surgical Quality Improvement Program. J Am Coll Surg 2004;199(4):531–537
13. Mahdi H, Goodrich S, Lockhart D, DeBernardo R, Moslemi-Kebria M. Prediction of surgical site infection in women undergoing hysterectomy for benign gynecologic disease: a multicenter analysis using the national surgical quality improvement program data. J Minim Invasive Gynecol 2014;21(5):901–909
14. Lim PC, Crane JT, English EJ, et al. Multicenter analysis comparing robotic, open, laparoscopic, and vaginal hysterectomies performed by high-volume surgeons for benign indications. Int J Gynaecol Obstet 2016;133(3):359–364
15. Winter ML, Leu SY, Lagrew DC Jr, Bustillo G. Cost comparison of robotic-assisted laparoscopic hysterectomy versus standard laparoscopic hysterectomy. J Robot Surg 2015;9(4):269–275
16. Bell MC, Torgerson J, Seshadri-Kreaden U, Suttle AW, Hunt S. Comparison of outcomes and cost for endometrial cancer staging via traditional laparotomy, standard laparoscopy and robotic techniques. Gynecol Oncol 2008; 111(3):407–411
17. Lau S, Vaknin Z, Ramana-Kumar AV, Halliday D, Franco EL, Gotlieb WH. Outcomes and cost comparisons after introducing a robotics program for endometrial cancer surgery. Obstet Gynecol 2012;119(4):717–724
18. Moawad GN, Abi Khalil ED, Tyan P, et al. Comparison of cost and operative outcomes of robotic hysterectomy compared to laparoscopic hysterectomy across different uterine weights. J Robot Surg 2017;11(4):433–439
19. Advincula AP, Xu X, Goudeau S IV, Ransom SB. Robot-assisted laparoscopic myomectomy versus abdominal myomectomy: a comparison of short-term surgical outcomes and immediate costs. J Minim Invasive Gynecol 2007; 14(6):698–705
20. Walker JL, Piedmonte MR, Spirtos NM, et al. Laparoscopy compared with laparotomy for comprehensive surgical staging of uterine cancer: Gynecologic Oncology Group Study LAP2. J Clin Oncol 2009;27(32):5331–5336
21. Seamon LG, Cohn DE, Henretta MS, et al. Minimally invasive comprehensive surgical staging for endometrial cancer: Robotics or laparoscopy? Gynecol Oncol 2009;113(1): 36–41

22. Walker JL, Piedmonte MR, Spirtos NM, et al. Recurrence and survival after random assignment to laparoscopy versus laparotomy for comprehensive surgical staging of uterine cancer: Gynecologic Oncology Group LAP2 Study. J Clin Oncol 2012;30(7):695–700

23. Estape R, Lambrou N, Diaz R, Estape E, Dunkin N, Rivera A. A case matched analysis of robotic radical hysterectomy with lymphadenectomy compared with laparoscopy and laparotomy. Gynecol Oncol 2009;113(3):357–361

24. Lim PC, Kang E, Park DH. A comparative detail analysis of the learning curve and surgical outcome for robotic hysterectomy with lymphadenectomy versus laparoscopic hysterectomy with lymphadenectomy in treatment of endometrial cancer: a case-matched controlled study of the first one hundred twenty two patients. Gynecol Oncol 2011;120(3):413–418

25. Abitbol J, Cohn R, Hunter S, et al. Minimizing pain medication use and its associated costs following robotic surgery. Gynecol Oncol 2017;144(1):187–192

26. Agarwal R, Rajanbabu A, Unnikrishnan UG. A retrospective evaluation of the perioperative drug use and comparison of its cost in robotic versus open surgery for endometrial cancer. J Robot Surg 2018;12(4):665–672

27. Barnett JC, Judd JP, Wu JM, Scales CD Jr, Myers ER, Havrilesky LJ. Cost comparison among robotic, laparoscopic, and open hysterectomy for endometrial cancer. Obstet Gynecol 2010; 116(3):685–693

28. Jonsdottir GM, Jorgensen S, Cohen SL, et al. Increasing minimally invasive hysterectomy: effect on cost and complications. Obstet Gynecol 2011;117(5):1142–1149

29. Hoekstra AV, Morgan JM, Lurain JR, et al. Robotic surgery in gynecologic oncology: impact on fellowship training. Gynecol Oncol 2009;114(2):168–172

30. Knight J, Talati A, Rao S, Escobar P. Trends in surgical training among gynecologic oncology fellows before and after the introduction of robotic surgery. Annual meeting in Women's Cancer; 2013. Los Angeles, CA, USA

31. Burkett D, Horwitz J, Kennedy V, Murphy D, Graziano S, Kenton K. Assessing current trends in resident hysterectomy training. Female Pelvic Med Reconstr Surg 2011;17(5):210–214

32. Smith AL, Schneider KM, Berens PD. Survey of obstetrics and gynecology residents' training and opinions on robotic surgery. J Robot Surg 2010;4(1):23–27

33. Sculpher M, Manca A, Abbott J, Fountain J, Mason S, Garry R. Cost effectiveness analysis of laparoscopic hysterectomy compared with standard hysterectomy: results from a randomised trial. BMJ 2004;328(7432):134

34. Aarts JW, Nieboer TE, Johnson N, et al. Surgical approach to hysterectomy for benign gynaecological disease. Cochrane Database Syst Rev 2015; (8):CD003677

Index